SPEECH PATHOLOGY
AND
FEEDBACK THEORY

SPEECH PATHOLOGY

AND

FEEDBACK THEORY

Second Printing

By

EDWARD D. MYSAK, Ph.D.

Professor of Speech Pathology
Chairman, Department of Speech Pathology and Audiology
Director, Speech and Hearing Center
Teachers College, Columbia University
Fellow of the American Speech and Hearing Association
New York, New York

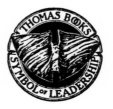

CHARLES C THOMAS · PUBLISHER
Springfield · Illinois · U.S.A.

Published and Distributed Throughout the World by
CHARLES C THOMAS • PUBLISHER
BANNERSTONE HOUSE
301-327 East Lawrence Avenue, Springfield, Illinois, U.S.A.
NATCHEZ PLANTATION HOUSE
735 North Atlantic Boulevard, Fort Lauderdale, Florida, U.S.A.

First Printing, 1966
Second Printing, 1971

With THOMAS BOOKS *careful attention is given to all details of
manufacturing and design. It is the Publisher's desire to present books
that are satisfactory as to their physical qualities and artistic possibilities
and appropriate for their particular use.* THOMAS BOOKS *will be true
to those laws of quality that assure a good name and good will.*

Printed in the United States of America
00-2

To Members of My Family

*Who have taught me so
much about talking and
who have done so much
patient listening ever
since*

PREFACE

THE MAJOR PURPOSE of this book is to specify the important practical and theoretical gains that may be derived from the translation of certain cybernetic concepts and terminology into speech behavioral terms. More specifically, it is believed that such a translation will contribute to the better understanding of normal speech processes, speech disorders, and remedial procedures for such disorders.

Since feedback theory ideas will be employed in the form and to the extent that they may make some contribution to the field of speech pathology, modifications of original meanings of certain feedback principles and terminology may sometimes occur. Related to this point, it would be well to mention here that physiologists considered the importance of reverberating tracts (feedback circuits) to human functioning long before the engineer applied the concept to the design of modern automatic control devices.

The book is divided into two parts: Part One is concerned with the area of speech behavior, and Part Two with the area of speech pathology. All the chapters are written from a "cybernetic" standpoint and all with the express purpose of extracting any new and worthwhile concepts that may arise from such an approach. Reference to standard speech pathology literature will be made sparingly and only when it is necessary to the development of some particular point which serves the basic purpose of the book.

Materials for the text have come from books on servomechanisms; from other speech pathologists who have applied cybernetic principles to speech disorders; and from personal teaching, clinical, and research experience. It should be stressed that many of the ideas presented in the book still need to be supported by controlled studies and long-term clinical application.

It is believed the text could be used to good advantage in classes for advanced undergraduates as well as graduate students of Speech Pathology and Audiology. Speech and hearing clinicians who are no longer formal students, but who desire to keep abreast of new ideas in their field, should also find the material of interest. Further, the material should prove of value to students and professionals in the fields of general speech, linguistics, and psychology, as well as in various health-related disciplines.

The author wishes to extend his sincere appreciation to all those individuals who helped in the preparation of this work. Special thanks are offered to: Theresa M. Mysak, for her untiring proofreading; Joseph T. Mysak, for his excellent illustrations; and Gloria E. Ponce, for her fine typing of many drafts of the original manuscript.

E.D.M.

CONTENTS

Preface vii

PART ONE
SPEECH BEHAVIOR

Chapter

1. AUTOMATIC CONTROL SYSTEMS AND SPEECH 5

    Automatic Control Devices 5

    Physiology and Automatic Control 7

    Behavior and Automatic Control 9

    Altered Sensory Feedback and Effects on Motor Behavior 12

    Altered Sensory Feedback and Effects on Speech 13

2. SPEECH SYSTEM 17

    Speaking as a Multiple-loop Phenomena 17

    Internal and External Multiple-loop Speech Behavior 19

    Functional Components of the Internal Speech Loop 21

    Feedback Terminology 28

3. SPEECH DEVELOPMENT 34

    Audiovocal Feedback 34

    Audioverbal Feedback 37

    Oral Language Theory 41

    Facilitation of Speech Development 42

PART TWO
SPEECH PATHOLOGY

4. SPOKEN SYMBOLS 47

    • CNS Impairment and Language Symptoms 47

    • Oral Language Disturbances in Childhood 49

    Therapy Procedures 52

    Feedback Disturbances in Aphasia 59

5. TONAL GENERATION 63

    Phonocybernetic Theory 63

Chapter

Page

Audioregulation in Voice Therapy.............................. 65
Additional Phonocybernetic Therapy Techniques................. 69

6. TONAL MODULATION 71
 Normal Acquisition of Speech Sounds......................... 71
 Irregular Speech Sound Acquisition.......................... 73
 Therapy Stage One 76
 Therapy Stage Two 80

7. TONAL FLOW 84
 Developmental Sequence of Tonal Flow Regulation............. 84
 Symptoms of Irregular Tonal Flow........................... 86
 Forms of Irregular Tonal Flow.............................. 89
 Re-automatization Therapy Procedures 93

Appendix: Logocybernetics and Behavior...................... 99

Index 107

SPEECH PATHOLOGY
AND
FEEDBACK THEORY

Part One
SPEECH BEHAVIOR

Chapter One

AUTOMATIC CONTROL SYSTEMS AND SPEECH

ORAL COMMUNICATION is one of the highest forms of behavior of which the human being is capable; consequently, a problem in oral communication may be considered as one of the most serious handicaps that a human can experience.

Since it is estimated there are upwards of ten million individuals with speech and hearing problems in the United States, the task of the field of Speech Pathology and Audiology is a prodigious one. In order to cope with the problem, increased research of speech and hearing processes and their disorders, and expanded and improved professional training programs are goals that must be achieved. However, because of the complexity of speech and hearing behavior such goals will not be gained easily or quickly.

Therefore, it behooves all those individuals associated with the field of Speech Pathology and Audiology to be alert to, and to take advantage of, all opportunities that may serve to hasten progress in any aspect of the field. In this connection, it has become manifest to the author, as well as to many authorities in the field, that the science of cybernetics, which was developed by Wiener (1948), contains concepts and language which, upon their translation into speech terms, can make significant theoretical and practical contributions to the field of Speech Pathology. The specific purpose of this book, then, is to attempt an initiatory translation of certain feedback concepts and language into terms related to speech behavior, speech disorders, and speech therapy.

In order to prepare the reader for the discussion of speech behavior from a cybernetic standpoint, the remaining sections of this chapter will present a general introduction to automatic control systems, followed by a discussion of certain physiological and behavioral mechanisms which act in cybernetic-like fashion, and, finally, a brief review of literature dealing with the effects of altering sensory feedback on motor speech behavior.

AUTOMATIC CONTROL DEVICES

Servomechanism is a word derived from the Latin servus or slave and therefore describes a slave system. The concept, as it prevails in the field of engineering, involves devices that automatically operate and control various kinds of machines, instruments, or appliances. Mechanisms providing automatic control may be divided into open and closed-loop control systems, according to Brown and Campbell (1948). This book will draw information almost exclusively from the latter type of control system, since it is to this type that the speech system will be compared. However, it is believed that a discussion of both kinds of goal-directed machines, and the principles upon which they operate, will serve to elucidate the total concept of automatic control.

Open-loop Control. Open-loop systems describe devices which carry out a series of operations in a certain prescribed manner and which do not possess the potential for changing their operations in instances where the results are not those desired. Time-operated traffic lights and timing mechanisms in various home appliances serve as good illustrations of this type of automatic control.

In the case of the electric toaster, once the timer has been set and the bread depressed, the heating and bread-raising mechanisms will be turned off and on, respectively, regardless of whether the bread has been toasted in exactly the manner desired. That is, you may set your toaster in the usual way, but because the bread you place into the toaster may be different from its usual quality it may begin to overtoast. However, because the toaster is an open-loop system, this event will have no effect on the heating mechanism and it will continue to heat the bread until the end of the pre-set duration time and very likely produce a burned piece of toast. Another example of an open-loop system is the automatic washing machine. The washing cycle of the machine ceases at the pre-set time irrespective of whether the clothes have been adequately cleaned or not. Electric dryers, coffee pots, dishwashers, and so forth, also belong in the open-loop category.

The important point to remember here is that such open-loop devices do not contain mechanisms which measure the machine's output and which can make machine adjustments if the results are not those desired. This is in contrast to the next class of automatic control devices known as closed-loop control systems.

Closed-loop Control. Closed-loop systems are different from open-loop systems inasmuch as they are error sensitive, error measuring, self-adjusting, goal-directed mechanisms. These systems operate to control the machine of which they are a part. They feed back into the machine information pertaining to its performance and, thereby, effect automatic corrections whenever error-performance signals are received. Familiar mechanisms of this type include home heating, water heating, and refrigerator thermostats. Industrial automation mechanisms, aircraft automatic pilot devices, and missile and torpedo guidance systems are also closed-loop control mechanisms.

To elaborate on the example of automatic home heating, once the thermostat has been set at a certain temperature level, the servomechanism assumes control over the furnace and will turn on or switch off the furnace depending on how close the room temperature approaches the pre-set desired temperature. As an example of missile guidance systems, let us consider a heat sensitive air-to-air missile. Once the missile is released by the attacking pilot, it goes forward, makes trajectory errors, and automatically corrects and adjusts its path; all as a function of receiving error signals from its heat sensors which react to the heat emanating from the engine exhaust of the target plane. This process causes the goal-oriented missile to follow and to eventually strike its target.

Next, certain aspects of human physiology will be discussed from the standpoint of automatic control.

PHYSIOLOGY AND AUTOMATIC CONTROL

Many activities of the human organism involve error-sensitive, error-measuring, self-adjusting functions which are analogous to servomechanistic operation. Mechanisms which quickly come to mind are those responsible for physiological homeostasis. Stabilization of vital functions of the organism makes it possible for other parts of the organism to engage in activities which are on higher levels. In other words, when lower sections of the brain care for physiological needs, higher sections are allowed to engage in intellectual pursuits such as observation, association, comparison, and evaluation. Such mechanisms control the constancy of temperature, water, sugar, calcium and oxygen contents, blood circulation, food intake, and so on. Brief descriptions of a few of these mechanisms will follow. It will be recognized that these physiologic controls are basically closed-loop control systems that operate on principles similar to electromechanical servomechanisms. More complete descriptions of these physiologic processes may be found by referring to Fulton's textbook (1955).

Thermal Equilibrium. The hypothalamus may be thought of as a physiological thermostat which regulates heat production and heat loss. It does so by influencing the somatic and visceral motor neurons of the brain stem and spinal cord. It appears that the anterior hypothalamus has the function of protecting the creature against overheating, while the posterior hypothalamus protects the creature against cooling. The peripheral mechanism for thermostasis includes the thermal sensitive endings of the skin and mucous membranes which react to environmental temperature changes. In the presence of cold, the physiologic thermostat, in order to increase the total amount of heat contained within the body, excites mechanisms which cause the cessation of sweating, the initiation of shivering, pilo-erection, and vasoconstriction. Conversely, in order to dispose of body heat in the event of heat exposure, mechanisms are excited which cause muscular relaxation, sweating, and cutaneous vasodilation.

This body heat regulation process may be described in servomechanistic terms as follows: Error signals in the form of excessive or reduced body heat are sent to a corrector device in the hypothalamus which subsequently excites appropriate portions of the nervous system. This excitation results in certain muscular and secretory activities which cause the loss or retention of body heat. Such feedback and correction continues until the system stabilizes and no thermal error signals are received.

Respiratory Regulation. Carbon dioxide is considered to play a major role in the regulation of respiration. Respiratory rates increase as the proportion of CO_2 in the air increases. Apparently CO_2 acts upon the final efferent neurons of the respiratory center and this causes an increase in the number of neurons that fire, as well as an increase in the frequency and duration of their discharge.

Respiratory regulation processes, then, also seem to have a servomechanistic character. Error sensitive receptors report errors, in the form of excessive CO_2 content in the air, to the control center in the medulla; the corrector device in the medulla then excites the nervous system in ways which appropriately decrease or increase respiratory activity.

Hormonal Balance. The very function of the endocrine glands is autoregulatory in nature. Elevation of the blood sugar level, for example, is a stimulus which causes the secretion of insulin which, in turn, facilitates the elimination of sugar from the blood. Whereas, a reduction in sugar level is a specific stimulus for the secretion of epinephrine which enhances the release of sugar from the liver. Another example is the regulation of the rate of secretion of the trophic hormones of the pituitary body by the circulating level of secretions of their target organs. It appears that deficiency of the gonadal, thyroid, or adrenocortical hormones causes an increase in the rate of secretion of the pituitary hormones controlling these organs and tends to increase the rate of release of the former and to restore the normal hormonal balance. Conversely, an excess of gonadal, thyroid, or adrenocortical hormones appears to depress the secretion of the respective trophic hormones of the pituitary.

Physiological error sensitive, self-adjusting mechanisms are rather clearly demonstrated in the function of the glandular system.

Blood Pressure Regulation. Automatic control mechanisms are also apparent in the regulation of blood pressure. For example, in response to strenuous exercise, hemorrhage, or very high temperature, acute renal vasoconstriction occurs and the blood flow to the kidneys is decreased making more blood available for circulation to areas where the need is more important.

Water Balance. Because of the continuous loss of water by evaporation and excretions, there is a need to maintain a normal water balance in the body. This is done in the following manner: A reduction in water content in the body results in dehydration of localized cells in the hypothalamus which gives rise to the experience of thirst. Thirst experience then motivates the organism to seek and consume water and thereby maintain its water balance.

Servomechanistic characteristics are again reflected in this sequence of events. This series of examples of physiological control mechanisms concludes with a description of automatic control and brain rhythms.

Brain Rhythms. Portions of a book by Walter (1953) describe the operation of certain kinds of automatic, goal-directed mechanisms located within the brain. To cite two examples: There seems to be a correlation between visual images and brain alpha rhythms (8 to 13 cycles per second), and between pleasure feelings and brain theta rhythms (4 to 7 cycles per second). Relative to alpha rhythms, when most normal individuals close their eyes while electroencephalograms are being made alpha rhythms are generated. These rhythms are considered to be the brain's scanning mechanism seeking visual stimuli. In the case of theta rhythms, it has been found that such rhythms are generated in many individuals upon the cessation of pleasant sensations. Again, the brain appears to be scanning, but this time for pleasant stimuli.

Along these lines, Wiener (1948) discussed the possible pertinence of the cybernetic approach to neuropathology. He believed there was value in viewing certain losses of motor control from this standpoint and considered that knowledge concerning servomechanism malfunctioning might serve to offer clues relative to neurological malfunctioning.

BEHAVIOR AND AUTOMATIC CONTROL

The principles implicit in the theory of automatic control systems may be extended beyond electromechanical devices and physiological homeostasis to include various psychomotor and psychosocial phenomena; in this vein, Wiener (1956), and rather recently Rapoport (1959), a professor of mathematical biology, have already discussed the heuristic value of applying cybernetic theory to behavioral science.

Psychomotor Mechanisms. Wiener (1956) has made reference to certain human actions that fit under the category of psychomotor activity; the elaboration of one involving the driving of a car serves as a good example of servomechanistic psychomotor functioning. In driving, the mind decides first to drive the car from one geographical point to another. Once this decision has been made, the experienced driver releases his motor system, so to speak, and automatically turns the ignition key, presses the starter, engages the driving gear, depresses the accelerator, and adjusts the steering wheel. During cruising, there is continual adjustment of the steering wheel and regulation of speed to suit road conditions. All these movements during the course of driving are made almost completely in an automatic fashion.

The movements of the complex multi-muscle groups involved in these acts could not be individually willed without seriously impairing the driver's performance level, or at worst, making it impossible to drive.

A successful driving trip entails therefore: the selection of a geographical goal; the initiation of movement toward the goal by activating the vehicle with a series of complex automatic motor acts; the continual reception of visual, auditory, tactile, and proprioceptive feedbacks arising from road conditions and car movements; the continual correction of course based on these feedbacks; and, finally, the arrival at the intended destination. Cybernetic characteristics of input, output, error measuring and correcting are apparent. Similar automatic guidance mechanisms are also apparent when operating machinery such as sewing machines, lathes, and so forth, and also when participating in sports such as baseball, football, and swimming; in all these cases, the automatic guidance systems allow the higher 'thinking brain' to operate while the lower 'doing brain' handles the actual motor tasks; for example, as in speaking to a passenger or reading road signs while driving, or as in planning what you would like to do the next day while swimming.

Psychosocial Mechanisms. In a recent book (Maltz, 1960), a plastic surgeon, indicates how important the knowledge of psychology is to the plastic surgeon. He states that when one is involved in changing an individual's face or physical image he more often than not will also alter the individual's personality and behavior to varying degrees. In this connection, awareness of self-image psychology has been of special interest to Maltz and he believes that knowledge of cybernetic theory aids in the understanding of this school of psychology. He believes further that many of the principles involved in cybernetic theory may be utilized in helping to understand, and possibly to change human behavior. Maltz reports that the science of cybernetics views the subconscious mind as not a mind at all, but rather as a goal-striving servomechanism consisting of the brain and nervous system which is used and directed by the mind.

In terms of self-image psychology and cybernetic theory, if an individual feeds negative beliefs, attitudes and interpretations, or negative data, into his internal mechanism, he creates a negative self-image such as inferior, incapable, ugly, or undeserving. This data is then stored and eventually comes to represent a negative type of input and hence encourages a negative output. For example, if an individual convinces himself that he will fail in a certain task, these data are received by the impersonal goal-directed servomechanism which then creates the appropriate failure goal. The mechanism then tends to lead the individual toward his expected failure goal. However, if the process is reversed and positive data are fed into the mechanism which, in turn, creates positive expectations, the chances that a success goal will materialize are much greater. Throughout his book,

Maltz presents many examples of these mechanisms in operation; these examples fell into at least the following two categories.

Personality. Experiences with various patients and with various reports have caused Maltz to believe that a high correlation exists between type of self-image and type of behavior. Following are selected examples from these experiences and reports: (1) A boy with large ears who was often ridiculed, and whose self-image was consequently affected, was considered "moronic" and behaved accordingly. However, once his ears had been corrected and his self-image changed, his true potential as an alert and bright boy emerged. (2) In contrast, Maltz describes a girl who was extremely self-conscious because of an unattractive nose. After the nose had been corrected, she continued to behave as in the past because of an inability to adjust her self-image regardless of her changed and now attractive face. (3) At a certain VA hospital, a group of mental patients was asked to answer items on a personality test as though they were well-adjusted individuals. Three-fourths of the men returned improved performances over previous tests and also began to show concomitant positive behavioral changes; that is, because they had to imagine themselves as normal and well-adjusted, many of them began to feel and act like well-adjusted individuals.

Skills. Synthetic experience or imagination exercise also appears to have an effect on our subconscious mind. Again, selected illustrations from Maltz's book follow: (1) Three groups of students were involved in an experiment on the effects of mental practice in improving skill in basketball throws. One group did not practice at all; the second group actually practiced for twenty minutes a day for twenty days; the third group spent a similar amount of time imagining throwing and correcting throws. At the end of the experiment, the "no practice" group showed no improvement; however, the "actual practice" and the "imaginative practice" groups showed a 24 per cent and a 23 per cent improvement in scoring, respectively. (2) Another example cites how a relatively obscure chess player defeated a world champion by practicing positive chess in his mind for a period of three months. (3) A world famous pianist is reported to dislike practice and, therefore, seldom practices for any appreciable time at the actual keyboard. The pianist has revealed, however, that he practices in his head. (4) A famous golfer has reported that he mentally rehearses each golf shot before he makes it. He indicates that he makes the shot perfectly in his imagination and then depends on his muscle memory to carry out the actual shot just as he has imagined it. (5) Napoleon was also said to be a great student of imagination practice. He has been described as practicing soldiering in his imagination many years before going on the actual battlefield.

All these examples imply that when a person feeds positive data into his mind's servomechanism he thereby increases the chances of the mind's automatic guidance system for actualizing his positive goals.

Before concluding this section, it should be mentioned that Strauss and Kephart (1955) have also made interesting use of a cybernetic approach in discussing perceptual and behavioral disturbances in brain-injured children.

ALTERED SENSORY FEEDBACK AND EFFECTS ON MOTOR BEHAVIOR

Following are reports of the effects on motor behavior when certain sensory feedbacks are experimentally altered.

Chase and others (1961) reported on the effect or altering various sensory feedbacks on keytapping motor tasks. Keytapping performances (tapping a key at a specific rate and with a specific amount of pressure) were studied under conditions of decreased auditory feedback (auditory masking); decreased visual feedback (tapping hand screened from view); vibration (vibrators applied to arm to mask proprioceptive feedback); digital block of tapping finger; and a combination of all four conditions. They found that significant changes in rate and intensity of tapping resulted under conditions of decreased auditory feedback, vibration, and the combined condition. A second part of the study was concerned with the effects of different delayed sensory events on keytapping. The five conditions of delayed sensory feedback employed included: delayed auditory, visual, and tactile feedbacks; all three delayed events presented simultaneously; and the latter condition repeated with a digital block of the finger. The findings revealed no marked alteration of the motor task described. However, highly significant changes occurred under delayed sensory feedback when a more complex keytapping pattern was attempted. All delay conditions produced changes characterized by increased intensity and decreased rate of tapping.

Recent studies of the effects of delayed visual feedback (Smith, 1962) on certain visually-controlled motor tasks have been conducted by making use of videotape recorders. The procedure is as follows: a subject attempts to draw a picture while standing before the monitor of a closed-circuit television system. A curtain is hung between the subject's eyes and hand so that he can see the performance of his hand only by watching the image of his own hand movements on the monitor screen. The delay in visual feedback is accomplished by having the television camera register the hand performance; having the images recorded by means of a videotape recorder; and then playing back the images on the monitor screen after a short delay. As a result of such a delay in visual feedback, the motion pattern of the hand becomes inaccurate and disorganized and the individual may show emotional disturbances and loss of motivation.

The above studies point up the significant role played by sensory feedback in the control of voluntary movement.

ALTERED SENSORY FEEDBACK AND EFFECTS ON SPEECH

Almost exclusively, the research on the application of cybernetic principles to speech production and control has been involved with the effect of alterations in auditory feedback upon various aspects of speech output. Studies have explored the differential effects on speech of synchronous as well as delayed and accelerated speech feedback changes; and the findings have tended to give weight to the concept that speech production and control mechanisms have characteristics which are similar to servomechanisms. Even though such research has been conducted for only a relatively few years, the amount of literature is already considerable; however, for purposes of this section, allusions will be made to only a few selected studies.

Synchronous Speech Feedback. Black (1954) has reported that voice level varies inversely as the voice level of an individual's personal voice feedback changes. For example, if an individual's voice is either amplified or attenuated by electronic means, his voice level is returned from the environment differently, in terms of loudness, and he will therefore adjust the level of his voice accordingly. The effect of auditory masking may also be cited here. Hanley and Draegart (1949) noted that when individuals speak in the presence of noise, the voice level is directly influenced by the loudness of the noise. From a clinical standpoint, the introduction of masking noise and the concomitant effect on voice level has been used as a test of functional hearing loss under the name of the familiar Lombard Test. In addition, it is often noticed that individuals with conductive hearing losses, whereby the person perceives his voice as louder than it actually is, often speak with reduced loudness; whereas, individuals with sensorineural losses, whereby the person perceives his voice as softer than it actually is, often speak with increased loudness.

In light of this foregoing data, it is apparent that the ear is an important mechanism for adjusting phonatory behavior. Therefore, the auditory mechanism, in addition to its speech reception function, also possesses the property of a speech control system.

Before beginning the next portion of this section of the chapter, a useful reference may be made to other than auditory feedback phenomena. Here we will call on the reader's memory of certain dental experiences. Oral anesthesia, induced by an injection of novocain, may reduce touch, pressure, and movement sensations associated with tongue and other articulatory activity, and this condition may cause the dental patient to experience deterioration in his articulatory accuracy until the effects of the novocain wear off. This rather common dental experience points up the importance of sensory feedback other than auditory to speech production and control.

Along these lines, McCroskey (1958) conducted two experiments, parts of which involved disturbing tactile-kinesthetic feedback during speech production. He found that by anesthetizing the articulators, significant disturbance in articulation could be produced. He concluded that auditory feedback was essential in monitoring the duration and rate of speech, while tactile-kinesthetic feedback was essential in monitoring articulatory accuracy and intelligibility. In another investigation, Klein (1963) studied the effects on speech when auditory, tactile and combined auditory-tactile feedbacks were disrupted. Masking noise was used to disrupt the auditory feedback and a topical anesthesia was used to disrupt the tactile feedback (without disturbing kinesthesia). One finding revealed that disturbance of the tactile feedback alone caused articulatory changes. A recent study by Ringel and Steer (1963) investigated the effects of oral region tactile alterations in isolation or in interaction with auditory disturbances on speech performance. One finding indicated that anesthetizing the articulators caused a greater degree of articulatory disturbance than did auditory masking. These studies support the concept that automatic control over the articulators will be disturbed when certain touch, position, and movement sensations are either eliminated or reduced in intensity.

Delayed Speech Feedback. Various researchers have studied the effects on speaking when there is an interference in speech feedback transmission from an individual back to the same individual; or, in other words, where there is an electronically-induced retardation in the air-conducted return of a speaker's voice to his own ears.

Most investigators (Atkinson, 1952; Black, 1950; Lee, 1951; Tiffany and Hanley, 1952) have found that under conditions of delayed auditory feedback, vocal changes, such as increased intensity, slower rate, and rhythm breaks similar to stuttering, may be observed. Additionally, one study by Fairbanks and Guttmann (1958) indicated that under speech feedback delay, articulatory disturbance was the primary effect and that rises in vocal sound pressure level and fundamental frequency were indirect effects.

Accelerated Speech Feedback. Peters (1954) reported that upon accelerating the air-conducted return of a speaker's voice to his own ears, speaking rate was increased; while Dolch (1954) reported that feedback acceleration in combination with the feedback being transmitted to the ears 180 degrees out-of-phase to the signal emitted at the mouth encouraged harshness of voice, a slower rate, and increased intensity in the subject's vocal performance.

All these studies accentuate the speech control property of the auditory system and reveal that when experimentally-induced disturbances in the function of the auditory mechanism occur, various speech production disturbances also occur.

In short, this section presents research and clinical data which support the concept of the servomechanistic-like behavior of the speech system; at the same time, it reveals how much more experimental exploration remains to be done in this area.

The translation of cybernetic concepts into terms of speech behavior, speech disorders, and speech correction constitutes the subject matter of the remaining chapters of the book.

SUMMARY

1. The important theoretical and practical contributions to speech behavior and speech pathology which may be derived from the translation of cybernetic concepts and language into speech terms is stated.

2. Servomechanisms are defined and described. Definitions and examples of open-loop and closed-loop servosystems are presented. Emphasis is placed on the discussion of closed-loop systems, since it is to this type of servomechanism that speech behavior is compared. Closed-loop systems are defined as error sensitive, error measuring, self-adjusting, goal-directed mechanisms. It is shown that such mechanisms appear operative in various human physiological and behavioral activities.

3. Finally, a review of selected literature based on the effects of altered sensory feedback on motor and speech behavior is presented.

REFERENCES

ATKINSON, C. J.: Vocal responses during controlled aural stimulation. *J. Speech Hearing Dis., 17:*419-426, 1952.

BLACK, J. W.: The loudness of sidetone. *Speech Monogr., 21:*301-305, 1954.

BLACK, J. W.: The effect of delayed side-tone upon vocal rate and intensity. *J. Speech Hearing Dis., 16:*56-60, 1950.

BROWN, G. S., and CAMPBELL, D. P.: *Principles of Servomechanisms.* New York, Wiley, 1948.

CHASE, R. A., RAPIN, ISABELLE, GILDEN, L., SUTTON, S., and GUILFOYLE, G.: Studies on sensory feedback II: sensory feedback influences on keytapping motor tasks. *Quart. J. Exp. Psychol., 13:*153-167, 1961.

DOLCH, J. P., and SCHUBERT, E. D.: Study of body conducted side-tone. Univ. of Iowa, Signal Corps; Cont. DA-36-039 SC-42562, supplementary report, 6, 1954.

FAIRBANKS, G., and GUTTMAN, N.: Effects of delayed auditory feedback upon articulation. *J. Speech Hearing Res., 1:*12-22, 1958.

FULTON, J. F., Ed.: *A Textbook of Physiology.* Philadelphia, Saunders, 1955.

HANLEY, T. D., and DRAEGART, G. L.: Effect of level of distracting noise upon speaking rate, duration, and intensity. Tech. Rept. SCD 104-2-14, Contract N 6 or 1-104, T.C. 11, 1949.

KLEIN, D.: An experimental study of selected speech disturbances and adaptation effects under conditions of auditory, tactile, and auditory-tactile feedback interference. Unpublished Master's Thesis, Cornell University, June, 1963.

LEE, B. S.: Artificial stutter. *J. Speech Hearing Dis., 16:*53-55, 1951.

MALTZ, M.: *Psycho-Cybernetics.* New Jersey, Prentice-Hall, 1960.

McCROSKEY, R.: The relative contribution of auditory and tactile clues to certain aspects of speech. *Southern Speech J., 24:*84-90, 1958.

PETERS, R. W.: The effect of changes in side-tone delay and level upon rate of oral reading of normal speakers. *J. Speech Hearing Dis., 19:*483-490, 1954.

RAPOPORT, A.: Mathematics and cybernetics. In: S. Arieti, Ed., *American Handbook of Psychiatry, Volume Two.* New York, Basic Books, 1959.

RINGEL, R. L., and STEER, M. D.: Some effects of tactile and auditory alterations on speech output. *J. Speech Hearing Res., 6:*369-378, 1963.

SMITH, K. U.: *Delayed Sensory Feedback and Behavior.* Philadelphia and London, Saunders, 1962.

STRAUSS, A. A., and KEPHART, N. C.: *Psychopathology and Education of the Brain-Injured Child, Vol. 2.* New York, Grune and Stratton, 1955.

TIFFANY, W. R., and HANLEY, C. W.: Delayed speech feedback as a test for auditory malingering. *Science, 115:*59-60, 1952.

WALTER, W. G.: *The Living Brain.* New York, Norton, 1953.

WIENER, N.: *Cybernetics.* New York, Wiley, 1948.

WIENER, N.: *The Human Use of Human Beings,* 2nd Ed. New York, Doubleday, 1956.

Chapter Two

SPEECH SYSTEM

IT MAY be recalled that closed-loop control devices were defined as systems which operate to control the machine of which they are a part. Specifically, these machines function on the basis of some type of input quantity or energy being introduced into the system; this, then, causes some type of machine action which results eventually in some type of output or product. A comparison of actual and desired outputs follows, and if there are any discrepancies, there is a feedback of error signals. These error signals are then combined with the input signal to form a corrected input and finally the desired output, and hence system stability is realized. This describes, in short, the error-sensitive, error-measuring, self-correcting characteristics of closed-loop systems. As further introduction to the discussion of the speech system as a closed-loop system, there is need to explain the distinction between single and multiple-loop systems.

Single-loop systems, as the term implies, refer to mechanisms having no subsystems operating within larger overall control systems. Multiple-loop systems, on the other hand, are complex mechanisms which have minor control loops or subsystems operating within main loops or larger overall control systems. With that brief explanation, and because the speech system itself serves as an example of a complex multiple-loop system, let us proceed to the discussion of the speech mechanism as a complex closed-loop system.

SPEAKING AS A MULTIPLE-LOOP PHENOMENA

The speech system may be viewed as a closed, multiple-loop system containing feedforward and feedback internal and external loops. Following are details concerning the internal and external loop aspects.

Internal Loop. This aspect is concerned with all those processes which may take place within the individual and which are responsible for speech formation and monitoring and speech production and monitoring. Seven processes may be recognized in the operation of this internal system. It should be stressed, however, that not all seven processes are necessarily engaged during any particular speech act.

1. Thought Propagation. Thought patterns are evoked by either external stimulation or evoked from within and may take the form of various types of images (although more often than not they take the form of inner speech).

2. **Word Formation.** The feeding forward of developed thought patterns to areas in the brain responsible for creating corresponding word patterns constitutes the word formation process.

3. *Thought Pattern-Word Pattern Comparison.* The thought pattern-word pattern comparison process describes so called inner speech where one checks on what one is about to utter. Not all speaking situations require such processing. However, when a speaker desires to utter something in just a certain way, or if one needs to be cautious in his choice of words, this operation may be engaged. Such inner speech monitoring represents one of the feedback loops which make up the internal aspect of the multiple-loop speech system.

4. **Word Production.** Actual word production occurs when impulses from the word formation area are fed forward activating the primary motor speech areas which, in turn, innervate the appropriate respiratory, phonatory, and articulatory musculature.

5. *Actual Word Product-Desired Word Product Comparison.* The operation of actual word product-desired word product comparison involves error scanning and measuring of the speech product; this activity ensures the articulatory accuracy of the speech output. Internal loops in this circuit may carry auditory, tactile, and proprioceptive signals back to the brain for processing. Speech product feedback monitoring describes the function of this operation.

6. *Word Product-Thought Pattern Comparison.* Concomitant with speech product feedback monitoring is speech content feedback monitoring. This feedback process ensures as high a degree of correspondence between thoughts and words as may be possible. Toward this end, the individual continually scrutinizes speech content output, compares it with his thoughts, and makes appropriate adjustments when necessary. The operation represents still another aspect of the internal, multiple-loop system.

7. *Speech Recycling.* If internal, multiple-loop activity is error-free, there is a continuing reduction of thoughts into words, or speech recycling.

Inspection of this internal, multiple-loop complex reveals at least two levels of activity: A higher "thinking level" devoted to thought and speech content monitoring, and a lower more automatic "doing level" devoted to articulatory (also rate, loudness, and voice factors) or speech product monitoring. It is because of these two levels of operation that an individual who misarticulates may not be auditorially aware of his error sound; that is, such an individual may be consciously engaged in speech content monitoring with his ears, but because speech product monitoring is usually left to tactile and proprioceptive channels, and is therefore on a less conscious level, he is not aware of his error sound.

External Loop. The feedforward aspect of the external loop of the multiple-loop speech system involves the directing of the spoken message at a listener; the feedback aspect consists of the evaluation of listener reactions by the speaker and the making of appropriate output corrections depending on the nature of these reactions. In order to complete the series of operations performed by the internal and external, multiple-loop speech system, three more processes must be added to those already discussed. These are: word product-listener reaction comparison; actual listener reaction-desired listener reaction comparison, and, finally, if all is error-free, speech recycling. Further information pertaining to these latter processes will be presented in the next section of the chapter.

In summary, then, considering both the internal and external loop aspects of the total speech system, the following ten operations may be recognized during a full cycle of speech behavior: (1) Thought propagation; (2) Word formation (feedforward); (3) Thought pattern-word pattern comparison (feedback); (4) Word production (feedforward); (5) Actual word product-desired word product comparison (feedback); (6) Word product-thought pattern comparison (feedback); (7) Internal, multiple-loop speech recycling; (8) Word product-listener reaction comparison (feedback); (9) Actual listener reaction-desired listener reaction comparison (feedback); and (10) Internal and external, multiple-loop speech recycling.

INTERNAL, AND EXTERNAL, MULTIPLE-LOOP SPEECH BEHAVIOR

Next, an example of the operation of a multiple-loop speech cycle will be presented. Let us imagine speaking to an individual and attempting to recall a mutual friend's name:

First, an idea is generated which stands for the friend, for example, you may visualize the friend's face or some other characteristic (thought propagation).

Second, the idea of the friend automatically (and reciprocally) excites the appropriate word association which, let us say, is "Joan" (word formation).

Third, there may be feedback and comparison of the word with the idea or "inner speech" checking (thought pattern-word pattern comparison).

Fourth, once it is willed, the release of the word pattern automatically results in the excitation of the appropriate neuromuscular configuration and the word "Joan" is uttered (word production).

Fifth, there is automatic speech product feedback (auditory, tactile, and proprioceptive signals) monitoring or inspection for the articulatory accuracy of the spoken word "Joan" (actual word product-desired word product comparison).

Sixth, a concomitant speech content feedback monitoring occurs on an auditory basis, whereby the accomplished spoken word is checked with the idea that it is supposed to represent (word product-thought pattern comparison).

Seventh, if the system is free of speech product and speech content errors, it proceeds to process additional speech cycles (internal loop speech recycling).

In order to illustrate the error-measuring, self-adjusting nature of the internal loop mechanism, or corrective internal loop recycling, let us suppose that the spoken word "Joan," during the sixth operation, feeds back error signals into the speech system to the effect that the word "Joan" is not the correct name after all. This causes the system to automatically scan for a new word association for the thought pattern, and let us imagine that these recycling procedures result in the development of the new word product, "Jane." This new word product may now be observed to create speech system stability.

Eighth, the external loop becomes active as this new word product is directed at the listener for his consideration. Suppose the corrected word product "Jane" causes the listener to shake his head in a negative fashion, and that these negative signals are fed back to the speaker. The listener reaction may be due to the fact that the word "Jane" elicits a thought pattern of a person other than the mutual friend in question and this situation causes the automatic generation of negative signals from the listener (word product-listener reaction comparison).

Ninth, because the speaker seeks agreement from his listener, he carefully scans the reaction of his listener. And, as an example of external loop error measuring and self-adjusting, the error signals emanating from the listener are received and acted upon causing corrective recycling and the system may be noted to return to the original word product "Joan." This word product may now produce positive feedback signals from the listener (actual listener reaction-desired listener reaction comparison).

Tenth, when there are positive feedbacks from both speaker and listener, the speaker proceeds to reduce new thoughts into words and the conversation continues (multiple-loop speech recycling).

The foregoing example reveals that dynamic oral communication depends on the interaction of a series of automatic and reciprocal relationships within the many internal and external loops which comprise the multiple-loop speech system. It also brings to mind the principle of the unity of the multiple-loop oral linguistic circuitry; a principle analogous to that described by Meader and Muyskens (1959) in their discussion of the unity of the organism. Four aspects of the principle may be recognized.

1. Relativity. All parts of the internal and external loop oral linguistic circuitry are interrelated.

2. *Self-reflexiveness.* Every part of the circuitry tends to influence every other part.

3. *Nonelementalism.* No part of the total circuitry can be fully understood in isolation.

4. *Unitary Structure.* Understanding of each part of the total circuitry in its relation to the other is essential to the understanding of the total circuitry.

The principle has important theoretical and practical significance to the speech scientist and clinician. So often research or remedial procedures are conducted without consideration of one or another of its aspects.

Finally, returning to the speaking example, malfunctioning in any one of the ten operations described may reflect itself in some type of oral communicative disorder. Problems may develop from speech generation or feedforward sources, or from speech monitoring or feedback sources. Certain disorders, therefore, are suggested by speech system cybernation which are not now covered by our present systems of classification. Reference will be made to some of these problems in the second part of the book.

FUNCTIONAL COMPONENTS OF THE INTERNAL SPEECH LOOP

Detailed descriptions of the various functional components included in the internal loop of the speech system as well as the anatomical and physiological representations of these components will now be presented. A model of the internal loop has already been presented by the author in a journal article (Mysak, 1959); the model was an extension of one designed by Fairbanks (1954). Comparison of that model and its accompanying discussion with the present Figure 1 would reveal numerous changes. These changes have come about due to the availability of new data and also in the interest of simplifying and clarifying the expressed concepts.

Receptor. The receptor unit represents the first section of the internal loop. It is made up of three basic components which subserve the estimating function of the sensorium. This section processes sensations such as: radiant energy via the eye (receptor 1), sound pressure energy via the ear (receptor 2), and mechanical energy via the end organs of touch (receptor 3). Proprioceptive end organs (receptor 4) are not included, however, it is possible that proprioceptive sensations may also be utilized in speech reception in special cases. The eye and ear are commonly recognized as speech receivers, but it should be recognized that touch and secondary movement sensations can be associated with meaning also. For example, individuals without sight or hearing can learn to make meaningful associations by reacting to touch sensations arising from the act of writing in the palms of their hands; or by feeling the movements of the articulators of the speaker

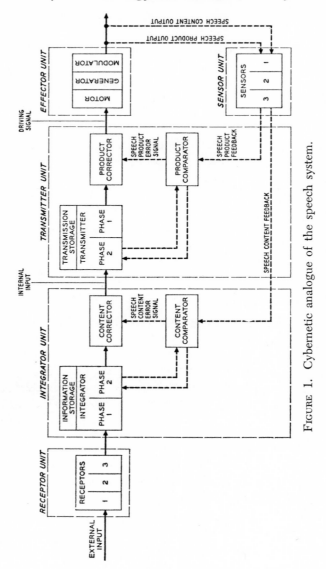

FIGURE 1. Cybernetic analogue of the speech system.

as they move and make certain contacts. It has been pointed out that such sensing of articulatory movements, as well as associated intraoral breath pressures, may also have remedial benefits when used with certain types of misarticulators, speech retardates, and aphasics. If the whole receptor unit were utilized in sending a word to a normal individual, he would receive every sensory dimension of which a word is composed. To illustrate: the word might be uttered while the listener listens to and watches the speaker, while he touches and feels the speaker's associated articulatory activity, and

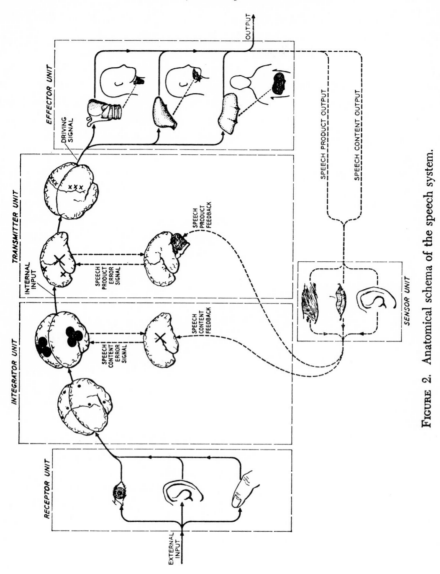

FIGURE 2. Anatomical schema of the speech system.

while he has his own articulators moved simultaneously through the various articulatory positions by the speaker.

It may be noted that Figure 2 uses a finger, an eye, and an ear to represent tactile, visual, and auditory reception. The cybernetic analogue (Fig. 1) places all the components within one unit to indicate the usual concomitant bisensory reception of such external speech stimuli.

Integrator. The second section of the system is called the integrator unit. Figure 1 shows that it is comprised of three basic components; the phase 1 integrator, the phase 2 integrator and the information storage component. Incoming information, in the form of speech sounds or other percepts, may be registered, retained, recalled, or responded to by this unit. Phase 1 integration involves the recognizing and the attaching of significance to incoming stimuli; phase 2 integration involves the interpreting and the elaborating of incoming stimuli, in addition to the forming of verbal and nonverbal response attitudes. Information retention is subtended by the storage component which retains or releases stored information upon command.

Phase 1 integration represents the perceptualizing process served by the many primary sensory areas in the brain which recognize and pattern incoming auditory, visual, and tactile stimuli. Phase 2 integration represents the conceptualizing process served by the many secondary sensory areas of the brain which further process the various incoming stimuli in the manner already described. Figure 1 also shows an error-measuring device existing within the unit. In the case of a speech response, this device compares the actual speech content with the prescribed speech content and determines the presence or absence of error performance. The concept of storage, or the recording of perceptual information by the brain, has been interestingly discussed by Penfield and Roberts (1959). They found that stimulation of certain portions of the temporal cortex during brain surgery on conscious patients resulted in vivid and complete re-experiencing of various past experiences by the patients. It would appear that something like a permanent registration of focused upon sights and sounds takes place in certain temporal lobe brain mechanisms.

An example of the operation of the unit should contribute to the understanding of its function. In normal speech reception, the receptor unit receives acoustical as well as visual events associated with articulatory activity. Phase 1 integration consists of recognition of the acoustical and visual events as significant sound and sight stimuli which should be attended to, further processed, and possibly stored. The latter two steps are functions of phase 2 integration. For example, someone tells you the time is five o'clock. During this utterance, you recognize the spoken words as being pertinent auditory events and you attach meaning to them (phase 1 integration). Further processing of the utterance results in associations such as the utterance means: "It is time to go home;" or, "I cease working at that hour," and so forth (phase 2 integration). Storage of this information for future use may also occur. Additionally, the information represents a potential oral response, if, for example, someone should specifically ask you, "When do you stop working?"

Figure 2 illustrates that perceptualizing and conceptualizing processes are carried out by both hemispheres. In the cybernetic analogue, all components are placed together within one unit to indicate the interrelatedness of all the processes, thus illustrating the constant interaction among perceptualizing and conceptualizing processes and information storage; such interaction tends to enhance and refine these three functions of the integrator unit. Also present in the analogue's integrator unit is the speech content comparator and speech content corrector, or the integrator unit's corrector device. Figure 2 shows this device in the temporoparietal region of the left hemisphere. The speech content corrector device functions as follows: Once the integrator has selected a certain response, it presents the neuronal pattern or nervous arrangement representing the idea to the cortico-thalamic area, which is the phase 2 transmitter component of the transmitter unit (the next unit to be discussed). This presentation automatically activates a neuronal pattern of corresponding words. In addition, the signal also has the potential for keeping the word neuronal-pattern active even after it discharges its pattern of signals into the phase 1 transmitter component, or the primary motor areas along the Rolandic fissure. Consequently, information in the form of speech is being sent out while at the same time word neuronal-patterns representative of the information being sent persist somewhere in the temporoparietal area in the left hemisphere. Via the auditory mechanism then, the transmitted speech content is fed back to the temporoparietal area where actual speech content patterns are compared with intended speech content patterns. If discrepancies are found, or if changes appear desirable, there is scanning for different neuronal concept-patterns which, consequently, result in different neuronal word-patterns and hence different speech output.

Transmitter. The transmitter section also has three basic parts and hence at least three functions. As already stated, ideas or speech intentions issuing from the integrator unit automatically excite word patterns in the phase 2 transmitter component which, in turn, activate appropriate signals in the phase 1 transmitter component. Phase 1 transmission is responsible for exciting, simultaneously, the motor, generator, and modulator components of the effector unit which are actually responsible for producing the desired spoken words. In addition to these primary parts and functions, the unit also possesses a corrector device which operates as follows: The speech product comparator receives the input signals as well as the output feedback signals and determines the difference between the two; error signals, if present, represent the amount by which the command issued by phase 2 transmission has not been achieved by the effector unit. These error signals are then sent to the speech product corrector which combines error signal and input signal into a new corrected driving signal. The error signal also returns to the phase 2 transmitter component where it can trigger off the next command when the present output is error-free, or where it can hold the next command when the output contains error factors. This latter function represents a predictor potential existing within the speech product comparator (Fairbanks, 1954) which allows command signals to flow rapidly without feedback monitoring when error-free sound products are anticipated. A similar predictor potential may be considered to exist within the integrator unit. The last component in the unit is called transmission storage and represents the place where functional word patterns are stored. Another function of this component is activated when the individual becomes a listener and is receiving words; that is, words coming from a speaker activate corresponding word patterns in the listener's transmission storage section which, in turn, automatically excite associated ideas.

The phase 2 transmitter component may be considered to be the secondary motor speech area or cortico-thalamic unit whose cortical areas, according to Penfield and Roberts (1959), almost always are located in the left hemisphere. Broca's area, the supplementary motor, and the temporoparietal areas are said to comprise the unit—the latter area is considered the most important. The phase 1 transmitter component represents the primary motor speech areas found along the anterior portion of the central fissure. These areas are responsible for innervating the respiratory-phonatory-articulatory muscle complex which produces the spoken word. As for the error-measuring function during word production, Ruch (1951) has made statements about the activity of the cerebellum which have a bearing on this component. In terms of guidance of movements, he conjectures that the cerebellum could be seen as the comparator component of a servomechanism. He indicates that it may receive signals from the cortex which represent the prescribed movement, and proprioceptive feedback signals from the muscles which represent the actual movement. Upon comparison or error measuring, if a discrepancy is found between prescribed and actual movements, appropriate error signals are then sent to the motor cortex which, in turn, alters its signals to the muscles and hence reduces the error.

In terms of function, let us suppose a 21-year-old individual is asked for his age. His speech reception-response mechanism proceeds as follows: (a) Recognition of the auditory events produced by the interrogator by the phase 1 integrator; subsequent interpretation by the phase 2 integrator; and scanning of the integrator's information storage component for the thought pattern corresponding to the idea of personal age. (b) Upon selection of the appropriate thought neuronal-pattern, there is an automatic activation of the appropriate word neuronal-pattern in the phase 2 transmitter component. (c) The release of this word neuronal-pattern by the volitional mechanism excites the phase 1 transmission area along the Rolandic fissure which innervates the respiratory-phonatory-articulatory muscle complex needed to produce the word response, "twenty-one."

Figure 2 shows that the transmitter unit is comprised of the cortico-thalamic complex in one hemisphere, the primary motor speech areas represented in both hemispheres, and the comparator device represented, at least in part, by the cerebellum. In Figure 1, the analogue also shows an area for transmission storage which, as previously stated, represents the storage of word neuronal-patterns which the individual has developed and which are available to him.

Effector Unit. The effector unit is directly responsible for the production of speech events. It consists of three components: the motor, the generator, and the modulator. The motor is responsible for producing the air column which supports speech, the generator is responsible for vibrating this air column or for voicing, and the modulator is responsible for breaking-up the voiced air stream into particular articulatory units. The motor represents the respiratory structures; the generator represents the laryngeal structures; and the modulator the articulatory structures.

Figure 2 displays a larynx, tongue, and diaphragm to represent the effector unit. In Figure 1, the analogue shows all three components within one unit to indicate their interrelatedness.

Sensor Unit. The last section of the internal loop is the sensor unit. It has at least three components and is responsible for feeding back speech product and speech content data. Sensor 1 feeds back the auditory dimension of the sounds uttered; sensor 2 the tactile dimension; and sensor 3 the proprioceptive dimension. The unit may also include sensor 4 which represents the visual dimension; visual feedback would occur during mirror-speaking, for instance. Sensor 1 also feeds back the speech content.

To illustrate sensor unit functioning, let us suppose an individual has been asked for the name of his home town which is Syracuse. However, also suppose that he has just left the dentist's office where he received some novacain which is still in the process of wearing off, and thus he may be experiencing abnormal tactile and proprioceptive feedbacks. Under these circumstances, his response may be uttered as "Thyracuse." The sensor unit feeds back this speech signal to both product and content comparators. The content comparator will find the signal error-free since the name of the city is correct; however, the product comparator will find an error factor since the initial phoneme comprising the word product is incorrect. The product comparator then sends the error signal to the product corrector device for processing and this results in the immediate correction of "Thyracuse" to "Syracuse."

Figure 1 shows the sensor components combined into one unit to indicate their interrelatedness. Two feedback signals may be seen arising from the unit and they are the aforementioned speech product and speech content feedback signals. The sensor unit in Figure 2 is represented by pictures of: a muscle representing the proprioceptive end organs, lips in contact representing tactile end organs, and the ear representing the auditory system. When visual feedback is active, an eye may also be included here.

To summarize this section of the chapter, the speech system is made up of five basic units: the receptor, integrator, transmitter, effector, and sensor units. Both integrator and transmitter units include storage components as well as corrector devices. The system has two outputs, namely, speech product and speech content.

The final section of the chapter deals with definitions of feedback-oriented terminology.

FEEDBACK TERMINOLOGY

The following explanations of terms should contribute further to reader orientation to the remaining chapters of the book; more specifically, portions of the discussion will suggest the kinds of applications of cybernetic theory to speech disorders which will be found in part two of the book.

Positive and Negative Speech Feedback. When the speech mechanism is operating in a relatively error-free manner, positive feedback or correct-operation feedback may be said to prevail. Error-free speech content and error-free speech product indicates total positive speech feedback.

When the mechanism is not functioning properly, the system will receive error signals or negative feedback; these error signals will then automatically engage the corrector device which adjusts speech mechanism operation. All closed-loop devices achieve their goal by negative feedback. For example, a salesman who is attempting to make a sale watches the reactions of the potential customer. If the customer appears to be reacting in a negative way, the salesman may shift his approach and intensify his sales line; in cybernetic terms, he is reacting appropriately to the reception of negative feedback from the external loop aspect of his multiple-loop speech system.

Regenerative and Degenerative Speech Feedback. Regenerative speech feedback may be experienced when one is speaking to a listener who is obviously interested in or enjoying one's speech content. This type of feedback encourages the speech system to continue operating and perhaps even to increase its output. Conversationalists, teachers, actors, and so on, have all experienced such external loop regenerative feedback at one time or another.

In contrast to regenerative speech feedback, negative signals in the form of disinterested listeners usually cause degenerative speech feedback and the speaker may reduce his speech output or eventually cease speaking entirely. Both types of feedback, and their associated concepts, have a bearing on problems of stuttering, adult aphasia, as well as on childhood language disturbances. Implications for speech hygiene as well as remedial procedures should also be apparent. The chapters on oral language and its pathology will delve more deeply into the therapy application of the concept of regenerative speech feedback.

Attenuated and Amplified Speech Feedback. If some factor in or outside the speech system weakens or eliminates the flow of speech feedback signals, a state of attenuated speech feedback may be said to exist. In the case of certain stutterers who auditorially over-monitor their speech, or who expect their speech to contain negative auditory feedback, masking, by presenting noise to their ears and thus attenuating auditory feedback, may cause them to become fluent. Such feedback alteration techniques will be elaborated upon in the chapter on stuttering.

In contrast, intensification of the feedback signal may be referred to as amplified speech feedback. During remedial procedures, for example, auditory stimuli produced by the clinician or by the client himself may be amplified by electronic means. Amplification of tactile and proprioceptive feedbacks may also have important implications in articulatory and stuttering therapy and will be touched on in subsequent chapters.

Double, Multiple Speech Feedback. Double, multiple speech feedback occurs when an individual slave speaks. For example, such feedback is experienced when a client watches a clinician's lips closely, expects certain words will be uttered, and speaks simultaneously with the clinician in slave fashion; by such activity, he receives auditory and visual signals from the speaker via his external loop system, and auditory, tactile, and proprioceptive feedback from his own speech behavior via his internal loop system. Echo speaking, where the listener repeats words after a speaker, is a form of delayed double, multiple speech feedback. Slave or echo speaking will be shown to have certain therapeutic benefits in those chapters concerned with stuttering and language pathology.

Synthetic or Imagery Speech Feedback. Synthetic speech feedback involves the evocation of certain imagery. To illustrate, remedial synthetic speech feedback may be utilized by having a stutterer engage in long periods of fluent speech, or by having an articulation case practicing the correct sound, both with their mind's articulators, so to speak. Such imagery practice may exert a positive influence on the speech product corrector device as well as on the speech product.

Anticipatory Speech Feedback. A condition whereby a speech system expects certain feedback signals before they occur may be described as an anticipatory feedback set. When such a set can be established in an individual it tends to sharpen the functioning of the sensor unit and also the functioning of the comparator component of the corrector device. Techniques designed to induce such anticipatory feedback sets, therefore, have important remedial implications.

Reverse Speech Feedback. With reference to the automatic and reciprocal relationship between thoughts and words, it is conceivable that the imposition of a certain articulatory pattern by a clinician upon a client (e.g., by use of the moto-kinesthetic approach) may, by virtue of the tactile-proprioceptive feedback, activate associated word and hence thought patterns. Additionally, stimulating random articulatory movements or mouthings by the client may similarly result in spontaneous vocalization. Reverse feedback therapy techniques appear to have some value in language disturbances.

Shunted Speech Feedback. If a system output is associated with more than one type of feedback, as is the case in the multiple-loop speech system, and one feedback channel is eliminated, thus allowing the remaining channels to dominate the system, the feedback characteristics of the system may be described as having been shunted. For example, if an individual speaks without voice or with whispered voice, he may be said to have shunted his speech product feedback more or less exclusively over to the tactile and proprioceptive channels. Techniques in shunting speech feedback have therapeutic pertinence if a speech system has a feedback channel which contains some type of interference. An over-sensitive auditory channel, for example, may feed back error signals which are in reality so minor as to be better disregarded. This "negative" feedback then causes the corrector device to be engaged unnecessarily and speech automaticity is affected. As has already been pointed out, this appears to be the problem in certain stutterers. By desensitizing the offending auditory channel, or by shunting the monitoring function to other sensor channels, fluency may be re-established.

Zero Speech Error. The characteristic of an ideal control mechanism is that it maintains a zero error state within a system. Zero error signals are experienced by the speech system during periods when both speech content and speech product are completely satisfactory. This situation is not experienced too frequently, however, since a good many speakers are not entirely satisfied with the way they express their thoughts. That is, a large percentage of sensitive speakers, after having spoken, usually become aware of better ways of saying what they have just said.

Steady State and Transient Speech Error. Steady state error signals are signals which develop during routine operation of the speech system. To illustrate, when a speaker is engaged in routine conversation, he may be said to be experiencing steady-state error signals associated either with speech product or speech content; and during this time, the individual's corrector device may be processing familiar slight differences between desired and actual speech output.

In contrast, when a system is required to correct for a sudden variation in the input signal, a transient error may be said to have occurred. With respect to the speech act, transient error correction may be manifested during cross-examination periods on a witness stand, or during active debates or discussions where a pressing interrogator may cause the need for swift and radical shifts in speech content. Under this condition, a speaker may be noticed to "uh" more, or show other signs of oscillation while he attempts to make, and adjust to major corrections in speech output.

Infused Speech Error. With respect to speech therapy, it is often necessary to intentionally introduce an auditory error signal as a prerequisite to effective remedial work, since so frequently in cases of error-sound production the individual is not auditorially aware of his error. Such speech error infusion is needed because it is believed by some authorities that after individuals master articulatory skills they use tactile and kinesthetic monitoring channels almost exclusively and reserve the ear for receiving speech content from others and for personal speech content monitoring; and hence they no longer react to auditory error signals associated with particular error-sound productions. This monitor function transition has important therapy implications for articulation and voice cases.

Speech System Overdamping and Underdamping. In physics, damping refers to the progressive reduction in amplitude of oscillations. In terms of servomechanisms, an overdamped system is one that requires more time for correction but which possesses more system stability. Underdamping, on the other hand, describes a system which responds more quickly to errors but whose response is oscillatory. System stability and response time therefore are factors to consider relative to the degree of damping which may be desired for any particular device.

The concept of overdamping, with reference to speech behavior, may be translated in the following way: Some individuals in the course of a discussion in which they are attempting to indicate their agreement with a speaking partner, but where they are not sure of the partner's point of view, may very slowly and without much outward sign adjust their speech output so as to agree with him. As an illustration, suppose one is speaking with a superior about politics and would like to be on the so-called right side by adopting whatever views the superior may hold—at least, while the individual is in the presence of the superior. This individual may present topics such as states rights, labor unions, big business, taxes, and watch closely for signs which may indicate a traditional Republican or Democratic reaction. He then slowly adjusts his comments to come more in line with the view he thinks his listener holds. However, because of the nature of his particular speech system, the process may be so slow that the conversation may end before the speaker accomplishes his goal. This serves as an example of an overdamped system for speech content correction marked by a slow and steady adjustment of the speech output.

Underdamping, on the other hand, describes a speech system which attempts to make rapid shifts in output depending on error signals received from without. Returning to the example, let us suppose that the individual attempting to make the impression says, "I think that the President really had a sensitive decision to make relative to his criticism of big business, but possibly there was merit in his final actions." The speaker is casting about for a response and may quickly become aware of many negative signs coming from the listener. If the speaker's system is underdamped, he responds quickly to the negative listener reactions, but system stability may be affected and the utterance emerges as: "uh, uh, but, but, the way he stated his case certainly revealed bias."

The concept of speech system underdamping or over-correcting may have a specific bearing on the problem of stuttering. For instance, if a system is too sensitive to negative feedback or machine criticism, exaggerated oscillations or complete cessation of machine functioning may occur. Similarly, if an individual over-reacts to negative feedback from himself or from his environment, this speech hyper-sensitivity may cause speech system oscillation and fixation, or, in other words, stuttering.

Alloplastic and Autoplastic Speech Systems. Alloplastic processes describe those which are performed with the help of someone else; in contrast, processes that depend on the self and that are self-made are called autoplastic. An alloplastic speech system, therefore, is one which depends on the speech partner to initiate or maintain a conversation, while an autoplastic speech system is one which assumes the initiative and carries the conversation. An ideal speech system would be one which contains a proper balance of both alloplastic and autoplastic characteristics. A good speech clinician, for example, would be one whose speech system contained such a balance; at the same time, however, he should be able to manipulate these characteristics at will.

In terms of speech pathology, whether a particular aphasic's premorbid speech system was alloplastic or autoplastic might have an important bearing on his reaction to his loss of speech and, consequently, on his recovery potential. Further reference to this concept will be made in various chapters in part two of the book.

Internal and External Loop Scanning. Scanning describes that process by which a mechanism explores and selectively brings to attention those items which are appropriate for a particular problem situation. Internal loop speech scanning involves the examination of the information storage component for particular thought patterns; or, the examination of the transmission storage component for particular word patterns. External loop speech scanning describes the examination of the speech product or content of others. The importance of the scanning process to speech perception, production, and correction should be self-evident.

SUMMARY

1. The speech system is described as a closed, multiple-loop system containing feedforward and feedback internal and external loops. Ten oper-

ations are described as possibly taking place during a full cycle of speech behavior; these are: thought propagation, word formation, thought pattern-word pattern comparison, word production, actual word product-desired word product comparison, word product-thought pattern comparison, internal, multiple-loop speech recycling, word product-listener reaction comparison, actual listener reaction-desired listener reaction comparison, and internal, and external, multiple-loop speech recycling.

2. Descriptions of the various functional components of the speech system's internal loop are presented. Figures of a cybernetic analogue of the speech system and an anatomical schema of the system are also presented. The speech system is described as being made up of five basic units: the receptor, integrator, transmitter, effector, and sensor units.

3. Explanations and examples of the following feedback terms are given: positive and negative speech feedback; regenerative and degenerative speech feedback; attenuated and amplified speech feedback; double, multiple speech feedback; synthetic speech feedback; anticipatory speech feedback; reverse speech feedback; shunted speech feedback; zero speech error; steady state and transient speech error; infused speech error; speech system overdamping and underdamping; and alloplastic and autoplastic speech characteristics.

REFERENCES

FAIRBANKS, G.: Systematic research in experimental phonetics: 1. A theory of the speech mechanism as a servosystem. *J. Speech Hearing Dis., 19*:133-139, 1954.

MEADER, C. L., and MUYSKENS, J. H.: *Handbook of Biolinguistics, Part Two.* Toledo, Weller, 1959.

MYSAK, E. D.: A servo model for speech therapy. *J. Speech Hearing Dis., 24*:144-149, 1959.

PENFIELD, W., and ROBERTS, L.: *Speech and Brain-Mechanisms.* Princeton, Princeton Univ. Press, 1959.

RUCH, T. C.: Motor systems. In: *Handbook of Experimental Psychology,* S. S. Stevens, Ed., New York, Wiley, 1951.

VAN RIPER, C., and IRWIN, J. V.: *Voice and Articulation.* Englewood Cliffs, Prentice-Hall, 1958.

Chapter Three

SPEECH DEVELOPMENT

IN CHAPTER TWO the speech system was described as a closed, multiple-loop system containing feedforward and feedback internal and external loops. It was stated that during a full cycle of speech behavior as many as ten perceptual-linguistic operations might possibly be engaged. The operations include: (1) thought propagation; (2) word formation (feedforward); (3) thought pattern-word pattern comparison (feedback); (4) word production (feedforward); (5) actual word product-desired word product comparison (feedback); (6) word product-thought pattern comparison (feedback)—and if speech content and speech product are error-free—a continual reduction of thoughts into words follows; or (7) internal, multiple-loop speech recycling. And when the speech signals are directed at a listener, there are at least three more operations involved: (8) word product-listener reaction comparison (feedback); (9) actual listener reaction—desired listener reaction comparison (feedback); and, finally, if listener reactions are also error-free, (10) internal, and external, multiple-loop speech recycling. These, then, are the operations that a developing speech system should perfect if it is to become efficient in intra- and intercommunication.

The central purpose of this chapter is to offer ideas on how these operations begin, develop, and are refined and established in new speech systems. For numerous ideas, and for certain specific data on various developmental progressions cited with reference to oral language, the writer wishes to acknowledge his indebtedness to workers such as Sheridan (1960), Berry and Eisenson (1956), Myklebust (1957), Strauss and Kephart (1955), and Mecham (1958). The writer will also draw information from one of his previously written articles (Mysak, 1961).

Two major stages which may be recognized in the sequential development of oral language are the prepropositional and propositional stages; a discussion of these two stages follows.

AUDIOVOCAL FEEDBACK

This section of the chapter will describe the sequential development of audiovocal feedback mechanisms during the prepropositional stage of speech development.

Open Audiovocal Loop. During the first four to six weeks, the child's auditory response behavior consists of "startle" activity such as body stiffening, eye blinking, and possibly crying to unexpected loud sounds. At this time, whimpering behavior may also be noted to cease in response to a nearby soft voice, and "auditory staring" behavior may be manifested by the child's momentary immobilization of his eyes in response to the ringing of a small bell held closely to the ear (3 to 5 inches).

Vocalization at this time is usually in response to unpleasant interoceptive sensations and consists of crying and screaming; however, gutteral sounds may also be heard when the infant is experiencing contented moments. This type of vocalization has been designated as reflexive vocalization. Sounds heard during this period may include [i, ɪ, ɛ, u, ʊ, h, k, ʔ].

The internal audiovocal loop is considered to be open at this time since the infant gives no apparent indication of self-hearing. However, an infantile, external feedforward loop may be identified, since the child's cry or scream holds signal value for adults in the area and may cause them to feed or otherwise soothe the infant. A similar primitive, environmental feedforward loop may also be appreciated, since certain noises (e.g., voice, bell) may be observed to cause the child to cease or to begin certain motor activity.

Closing, Internal Audiovocal Loop. At about three months, the infant still shows startle symptoms to unexpected loud noises; will stare or smile in response to his mother's voice; and will stare in response to the rattle of a spoon in a cup or to the ringing of a bell (6 to 12 inches from the ear). "Auditory searching" behavior may be manifested by the child's side-to-side head movements in response to sound, and the beginning of "auditory localizing" may be noted by the turning of the child's eyes toward the source of sound. At about six months, localization behavior is developed and is manifested by the child's ability to immediately localize his mother's voice. The child may also respond differentially, depending on the tone of the mother's voice. Correct localization, with possibly some delay in response, can be evoked by stimulation with a rattle, cup and spoon, paper or bell (1 to 1½ feet from each ear).

It should be instructive to review for the reader, the sequential development of auditory behavior up to this point. First, unexpected sound caused nonspecific motor reactions (startle response), then, auditory stimulation, in order, caused: auditory staring, searching, and, finally, localization. This kind of progression is in keeping with the developmental principle of: progression from gross, undifferentiated behavior to fine, differentiated behavior.

Vocalization may be heard at three, and up to six months, in response to speech, or when the child is content. The child may be heard to coo, gurgle, snort, grunt, laugh, or chuckle in reaction to pleasant internal or external experiences. He may be heard to vocalize single syllables, for example, [ɡʊ, mə, bæ, kɑ]. This vocalization is often referred to as babbling. Other sounds heard at this time may include: [e, æ, oʊ, g, ɑ, ɔ, ə, j, m, p, b, w].

The closing of the internal audiovocal loop is indicated by the child's reaction to self-produced sounds (e.g., by his facial expressions), and by his making of sounds during pleasant moments. The infantile, external feedforward loop continues to develop since the child may now make sounds for the purpose of eliciting parental reactions. The developing, environmental feedforward loop is also apparent, since the child reacts to the speech and other sounds made by individuals in the environment.

Figure 3-A illustrates this closing of the internal audiovocal loop by using a dotted line to represent the internal loop; the developing, environmental feedforward loop between the infant and the speech model is also represented by a dotted line.

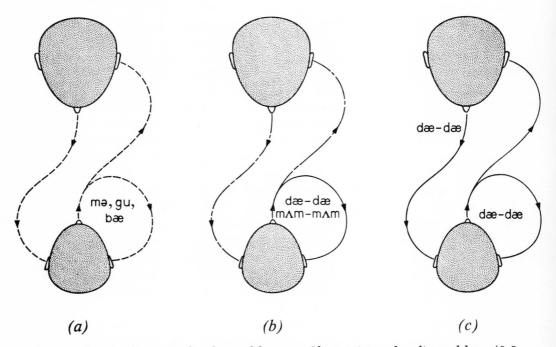

(a)   *(b)*   *(c)*

FIGURE 3. Development of audiovocal loops. a. Closing, internal audiovocal loop (0-6 months). b. Closed, internal audiovocal loop (6-9 months). c. Closed, internal and external audiovocal loops (9-12 months).

Closed, Internal Audiovocal Loop. At about nine months, the child may begin to show meaningful motor behavior in response to the calling of his name. He may also respond appropriately to words such as: "no" and "bye-bye." He may be observed to make immediate and correct localizing responses to instruments sounded at a distance of about three feet from the ear.

The infant may now shout to attract attention and may try to imitate play sounds made by adults such as: smacking lips, brrr, and so on. He may also be observed to repeat self-produced sounds or sound combinations. This type of vocalization has been called lalling. Sounds heard at this time may include: [t, d, n, l].

The repeating of self-produced sounds is indicative of the completed closing of the internal audiovocal loop. The continuing development of the environmental feedforward loop is evidenced by the child's reactions to certain spoken symbols, and his attempts at imitating various play sounds.

Figure 3-B indicates the closed, internal audiovocal loop by the solid line from the sound source to the child's ear. The further development of the external feedforward and environmental feedforward loops are illustrated by long lines followed by dashes emanating from both infant and speech model sources.

Closed, Internal and External Audiovocal Loops. At about twelve months, the child's auditory discrimination ability has reached the level where he recognizes and quickly responds to the calling of his name. He may also respond adequately to "no" and simple "give me" requests usually when associated with gesture. In addition, he may show by his movements and behavior that he understands a few words, such as family names, and may also respond appropriately to requests such as "come to Mommy." Immediate and accurate localizing responses to sound instruments may be observed when they are sounded at distances from three to four-and-one-half feet.

Vocalization has reached the level where the child may be heard to imitate sounds made by others. This type of vocalization has been called echolalia. Sounds heard at this time may include: [ʃ, s, z, tʃ].

The echolalic period is indicative of the closing of the internal and external audiovocal loops. Now the infant not only can repeat self-produced vocalization, but also imitates sounds produced by others. This, of course, is a significant step toward the eventual acquisition of true words.

Figure 3-C illustrates this development by the use of solid lines to represent the intact internal and external audiovocal loops from the infant, and also the environmental feedforward loop from the speech model.

This sequence brings the child to the end of the prepropositional stage of speech development. It should be emphasized that only the more readily observable auditory feedback sequence has been discussed. What precisely is taking place with respect to associated tactile and proprioceptive feedback developments is strictly a matter for speculation at this time. However, it is assumed that during the closing and closed audiovocal loop periods, associations are being formed between the auditory events and the accompanying articulatory touch and movement sensations which produce them.

AUDIOVERBAL FEEDBACK

The next section of the chapter will describe the sequential develop-

ment of audioverbal feedback mechanisms during the propositional stage
of oral language development.

Closing, Internal Audioverbal Loop. Up to about eighteen months, auditory discrimination capacity has reached the level whereby the child can
follow simple requests and directions. He may point to familiar persons and
toys when requested. He also obeys commands such as: "shut the door,"
"get your shoes." He also enjoys nursery rhymes and will show his own, or
a doll's hair, nose, mouth, and hand when requested.

At this time, his vocalization is characterized by the use of a great
amount of jargon. He may vocalize his desires at the table. He may also
echo the last word heard. Desired objects may be demanded by a combination of pointing and loud vocalizations or words. Attempts at singing and
joining in nursery rhymes may also be observed. As many as twenty words
may be recognized at this time.

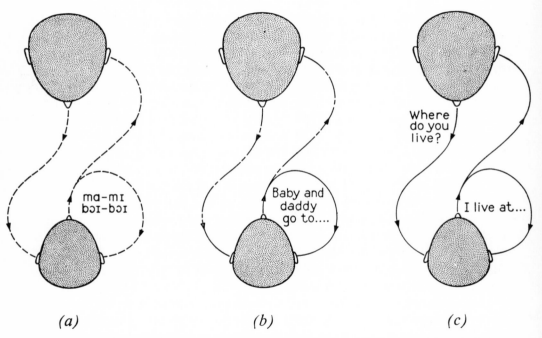

(a)   *(b)*   *(c)*

FIGURE 4. Development of audioverbal loops. a. Closing, internal audioverbal loop
(12-18 months). b. Closed, internal audioverbal loop (18 months-3 years). c. Closed,
internal and external audioverbal loops (3-8 years).

This period marks the beginning of perceptual-linguistic development.
The infant is very busy forming percepts, learning the associated heard
word-patterns, developing connections between the two, and, consequently,
using a few spoken word-patterns himself.

Figure 4-A illustrates this period by having the environmental, feedforward audioverbal loop represented by a dotted line, indicating limited comprehension of heard word-patterns; by having the child's external, audioverbal feedforward loop represented by a dotted line, indicating his limited use of spoken word-patterns; and, finally, by having the child's internal, audioverbal feedback loop also represented by a dotted line, indicating his developing ability to refine production and use of learned spoken symbols by virtue of auditory feedback monitoring.

Closed, Internal Audioverbal Loop. A significant factor in the development of meaningful oral language during the period from the utterance of the first true words to about the third year is the rapid increase in percept formation. And, of course, when all factors are equal, this growth in perceptualizing usually means growth in the use of heard and spoken word-patterns.

At about two years, auditory functioning has reached the point where the child will show, upon request, his hair, hand, feet, nose, eyes, mouth, and shoe. At about two-and-one-half years, he may enjoy simple stories read from a picture book; and by three years, he listens with interest to stories, and requests the repetition of favorite ones.

With respect to spoken word-patterns, the child at two years may use simple two-word sentences and may use as many as fifty recognizable words. He may also refer to himself by name.

At two-and-one-half years he may know his full name. Echolalia of word patterns persists. He uses I, me, you, and so on, in his speech and he may say a nursery rhyme. By three years of age, he may give his full name and sex and may carry on simple conversations. He names common pictures and verbalizes toilet needs. Basically, his external, audioverbal feedforward loop is characterized by the expression of wants and needs.

Important to the child's perceptual development during this period is his frequent asking for names of objects at about two years; his asking of questions beginning with "What?" and "Where?" at about two-and-one-half years; and his asking of questions beginning with "Who?" at about three years.

Important to our discussion is that during this period the child may be observed to accompany his activities with the words he is acquiring. He engages in what Piaget (1948, p. 9) called egocentric language. Piaget (1948, p. 40) also indicated that gestures, mimicry, and expressions are used as much as words at this time.

Hence, the child at two years of age may be observed to talk to himself rather continuously while playing. At two-and-one-half years, he may be found talking to himself during play concerning events happening here and now; and at three years, he still talks to himself in long monologues mostly concerned with the immediate present, including make-believe activities. This period from about eighteen months through three years is fundamentally a time when the child experiences internal loop perceptual-linguistic development. The child at this time uses speech to vocalize his perceptual processes (1955, p. 94). It is a period during which time the child, with the aid of speech, stabilizes, expands, and maintains an organized sequence to his perceptualization. Further, the word, during this period, actually represents the object and acts as a substitute for it.

Figure 4-B illustrates this phase in oral language development by symbolizing the child's increasing concern and interest in the heard words coming from the environment by a long line followed by a dash. The completed closing of the internal, audioverbal feedback loop is represented by a solid line, while the continuing development of the child's audioverbal feedforward loop is, as in the case of the environmental feedforward loop, represented by a long line followed by a dash.

Closed, Internal and External Audioverbal Loops. At four and five years of age, the child's auditory development enables him to listen to long stories. He is also interested in sharing his percepts, as well as in elaborating his own percepts by listening to the experiences of others.

In terms of spoken word-patterns, the child at four years of age may give a running account of recent events and experiences and may give his age and home address. He may also tell long stories. At five years of age, he usually gives his birthday. A good deal of his speech may be characterized by criticism, commands, requests, threats, and by questions and answers.

Important to the child's perceptual-conceptual development at this time is his frequent asking of questions beginning with "Why?" "When?" and "How?"; and his requests for the meaning of words. At five years of age, he may ask for the meanings of abstract words. From about five years to about seven or eight years, perceptualization development continues to the point where the percept is no longer limited to a representation of the object experienced. Strauss and Kephart (1955, p. 103) indicate that by virtue of perceptual selectivity, ". . . the perceptual image will become schematized and will lead to a general perceptual schema. Language at this point will become symbolic and, in interaction with the perceptual schema, will lead to thinking and reasoning as we know them in the adult." At this time, the word no longer merely represents the object but is a symbol for a differentiated perception. As symbolization develops, the child reflects the ability to analyze and synthesize elements from a number of perceptions into new wholes or conceptual units. Conceptualization begins at about seven or eight years, and it is at this time that the child's language resembles the symbolic intercommunication of the adult.

With closed, internal and external audioverbal loops, oral language development is completed. Inspection of Figure 4-C indicates this completed development by representing the environmental feedforward loop and the internal and external audioverbal loops of the child with solid lines. Now, there is rather easy comprehension of the speech signals coming from the environment, as well as rather easy formation, expression, and monitoring of verbal responses on the part of the child. It might also be pointed out here that this period marks the transition, in many individuals, from a basic audioregulation of speech product (articulatory events) to a basic tactile-proprioceptive regulation of speech product. Speech content monitoring remains, of course, the function of the auditory channel. More will be said about this monitor channel transition in the chapter devoted to articulation disorders.

The ten perceptual-linguistic operations referred to in Chapter Two may now be utilized by the child; of course, there will be further refinements in some of these ten operations as the child continues to mature. For instance, exactly how and when processes associated with thought pattern-word pattern comparison develop and refine can only be speculated upon at this time. Lack of organized information is also evident in connection with the operations of word product-thought pattern comparison, word product-listener reaction comparison, and actual listener reaction-desired listener reaction comparison. The latter operations no doubt develop to different levels of efficiency depending on the individual, and may be undergoing continual refinement well into adulthood.

Further, comparison of Figures 3 and 4 will reveal a parallel sequence with respect to feedback and feedforward loop developments; that is, it may be noted that during the prepropositional stage, the audiovocal loop development proceeds from a closing internal loop during the first six months of life, to a closed internal loop at six to nine months, to a closed internal and external loop at nine to twelve months. The propositional stage of oral language development follows the same sequence; that is, from closing to closed, internal audioverbal loops at twelve to eighteen months, and eighteen months to three years, respectively, to closed, internal and external audioverbal loops at three to eight years. The possible diagnostic and therapeutic implications of these audiovocal and audioverbal loop developmental sequences should not go unnoticed.

ORAL LANGUAGE THEORY

Related to the discussion of this chapter is Mowrer's (1958) rather well-known autism theory of language development which also may be interpreted from a feedback standpoint. The theory may be described simply in the following way: If a speaker wishes to have a child acquire a certain spoken word-pattern, the speaker must first come to represent positive emotional connotations for the potential speaker by providing pleasure sensations for the child during, for example, such actions as feeding, bathing, playing. Second, the speaker should produce a specific spoken word-pattern just before and as he confronts the child; this should be done until the speaker eventually evokes positive emotional feelings within the child by his word pattern alone. Third, during random vocalization, the child will experience a positive emotional feedback (self-stimulation) when he approximates the speaker's word pattern. Fourth, the child repeats the word approximation and refines it because he receives greater degrees of satisfaction from the feedback when he produces the word pattern more accurately. Fifth, the child retains the learned word-pattern because of the positive feedback received from the social approval of his utterance.

Figure 5 illustrates the above sequence of events in terms of feedback ideas, showing development of the various internal and external loops. Inspection of parts D, E, and F of Figure 5 reveals that, in Mowrer's explanation of speech development, we also have internal loop development preceding external loop development.

FACILITATION OF SPEECH DEVELOPMENT

It may be recalled that a section of Chapter Two was devoted to a discussion of feedback-oriented terminology. The last section of this chapter will elaborate on a few of those terms which are pertinent to the facilitation of speech development.

Regenerative Speech Feedback. Regenerative speech feedback is experienced by a speaker when his words are obviously being enjoyed and valued by his listener. Such environmental, external loop feedback tends to stimulate the speaker's speech system to continue operating and perhaps even to increase its output. Speech regenerative factors include: (1) a listener who exhibits close attention to what is being said, for example, by facial expression, eye contact, body posture, and so on, and whose attention does not wander; (2) a listener who does not threaten to intrude frequently into the speaker's flow of speech; and (3) a listener who does not quickly provide words for the speaker, or frequently correct pronunciation or articulation while the speaker is still verbalizing.

Alloplastic and Autoplastic Speech Systems. In Chapter Two, alloplastic speech systems were described as systems which depend on speaking partners to initiate and (or) maintain conversation, while autoplastic speech systems were ones which assume the initiative and carry the conversation. It would be well if new speakers could be guided so that: (1) a proper balance between alloplastic and autoplastic speech characteristics could be developed, and (2) the characteristics could be controlled and varied to suit the situation.

Toward this end, mature speakers should allow young speakers to initiate and carry conversations without frequently suggesting ideas to them or providing them with words for which they assume the child is searching. In keeping with the goal of proper balance of speech characteristics, mature

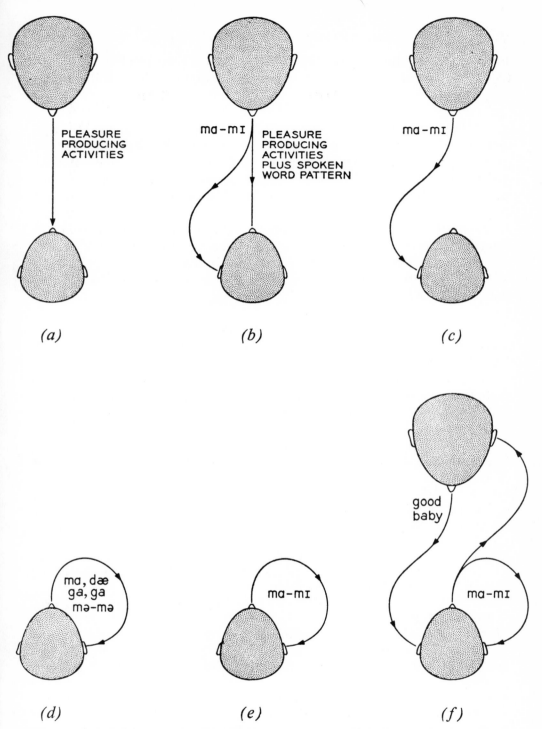

FIGURE 5. Feedback interpretation of Mowrer's autism theory of speech development. a. Positive sensations. b. Positive sensations plus hearing mɑ-mɪ. c. Positive sensations from hearing mɑ-mɪ alone. d. Self-elicited positive sensations from approximating mɑ-mɪ during random vocalization. e. Increased positive sensations from producing mɑ-mɪ more accurately. f. Retention of utterance mɑ-mɪ because of social approval.

speakers should also set good models as listeners so that the child may learn the value of, and appreciate the enjoyment from, being a good listener.

SUMMARY

1. Prepropositional and propositional stages of oral language development are discussed. The prepropositional stage includes the following sequence: closing, internal audiovocal loop; closed, internal audiovocal loop; and closed, internal and external audiovocal loops. This period covers approximately the first twelve months of life. The propositional stage of oral language development includes the following sequence: closing, internal audioverbal loop; closed, internal audioverbal loop; and closed, internal and external audioverbal loops. This period covers the time from the end of the first year until approximately eight years of age.

The similarity of the developmental sequences of both stages is evident, that is, closing to closed internal loops, followed by closed, internal and external loops.

2. Mowrer's Autism Theory of speech development is described from a feedback standpoint, and a similar sequence with respect to feedback loop development is noted.

3. The concepts of regenerative speech feedback and alloplastic and autoplastic speech characteristics are discussed with respect to their contribution to the development of a well-functioning speech system.

REFERENCES

BERRY, M. F., and EISENSON, J.: *Speech Disorders: Principles and Practices of Therapy.* New York, Appleton, 1956.

MECHAM, M. J.: *Verbal Language Development Scale: Manual of Item Definitions.* Philadelphia, Educational Publishers, 1958.

MOWRER, O. H.: Hearing and speaking: an analysis of language learning. *J. Speech Hearing Dis.,* 23:143-152, 1958.

MYKLEBUST, H. R.: Aphasia in children—language development and language pathology, and diagnosis and training. In: *Handbook of Speech Pathology,* L. E. Travis, Ed. New York, Appleton, 1957.

MYSAK, E. D.: Organismic development of oral language. *J. Speech Hearing Dis.,* 26:377-384, 1961.

PENFIELD, W., and ROBERTS, L.: *Speech and Brain Mechanisms.* Princeton, Princeton Univ. Press, 1959.

PIAGET, J.: *The Language and Thought of the Child,* 3rd Ed. London, Routledge, 1948.

SHERIDAN, MARY D.: *The Developmental Progress of Infants and Young Children.* London, Her Majesty's Stat. Off., 1960.

STRAUSS, A. A., and KEPHART, N. C.: *Psychopathology and Education of the Brain-Injured Child, Vol. 2.* New York, Grune and Stratton, 1955.

Part Two
SPEECH PATHOLOGY

Chapter Four

SPOKEN SYMBOLS

Since Chapter Four marks the beginning of the speech pathology part of the book, it would be well to remind the reader of a comment made in the preface which relates to the use of reference material. It was indicated that reference to standard speech pathology literature would be made only when it served the basic purpose of the book, which is: to increase insight into the symptoms of, and therapy procedures for, various speech disorders by examining them in the light of feedback theory. Hence, it will be assumed that the reader is already familiar with standard speech pathology literature.

Disorders in the comprehension, formation, and transmission of spoken symbols will be discussed in this chapter with special reference to the child who is experiencing difficulties in developing heard and spoken word-patterns because of CNS impairment. However, some reference will also be made at the close of the chapter to the adult speaker whose capacity to use oral language is affected because of aphasia. Further, this chapter will only consider disturbances in the fundamental language system, that is, disturbances in the understanding and use of spoken symbols. Disturbances in the use of written symbols, which are symbols for spoken symbols, will not be covered here.

In short, the specific purpose of this chapter is to interpret symptoms of language disorder, and to suggest remedial procedures for these symptoms, both from the standpoint of feedback theory.

CNS IMPAIRMENT AND LANGUAGE SYMPTOMS

It is believed that the following review of literature concerning CNS impairment and language symptoms will serve as useful introductory material to subsequent sections of the chapter.

Audition. Lewis, Strauss, and Lehtinen (1960, p. 126) describe the brain-injured child as one who has poor ability to organize and perceive auditory stimuli; and because of this problem, they may be observed to confuse speech sounds which are similar or they may reverse syllables within a word. In a similar vein, Ingram (1960), in reporting on the various symptoms in developmental dysphasia, stated that these children tend to make mistakes in properly arranging syllables to form meaningful words; they may omit or replace them with similar sounding syllables; or they may reverse or confuse their order. He also reported that these children have difficulty in comprehending speech especially during their early years. He remarked that even when these children learn to comprehend better, comprehension is still imperfect, and they may be noted to automatically ask that utterances be repeated. The more severely affected children are often observed to depend considerably on gesture and speechreading as a means of facilitating their comprehension of what is being spoken.

Words and Word Arrangement. With regard to problems with words and word arrangements, Strauss and Kephart (1955, p. 106) indicate that grammatical confusion is common even in those children who come from environments where good grammar is habitually used. Ingram (1960), in writing of children with developmental dysphasia, reported that ". . . Small words, especially those with only syntactical significance, are often omitted or mistaken . . . Grammar, sentence-structure and the ability to express complex ideas by an organized sequence of sentences are all impaired." Ingram also stated that the ". . . more severely affected patients are slow in acquiring words and in making phrases"—and that ". . . They tend to make mistakes in arranging the component syllables to make meaningful words, omitting some, replacing others by inappropriate speech sounds (especially those which sound similar), and reversing and otherwise confusing their order . . . Neologisms are frequent." Ingram also found that affected children suffer from word-finding difficulty as well.

Word Meanings. Many writers have reported that brain-damaged children frequently show a lack of meaning associated with their verbalization.

Strauss and Kephart (1955, p. 105), in commenting on the brain-injured child's perceptual difficulties, indicate that because of such difficulties they ". . . would expect that this child would frequently show a paucity of meaning attached to a given word." Lewis, Strauss, and Lehtinen (1960, p. 130) state, "It is not unusual to find that some brain-injured children are highly verbal. They seem to have good expressive language facility but some of this verbal facility may be imitative. The child may use words without being certain of their content. The percepts or concepts which the words represent may not be firmly evolved." Finally, Hagberg (1962), in describing a group of apparently "normal" children with minimal brain damage resulting from spontaneously arrested hydrocephalus, indicated that some of these children revealed symptoms of what he and his colleagues have called the "cocktail party syndrome." "These children are very sociable and pseudobright and love to chatter but usually do not know very much what they are talking about."

In the following section of the chapter, explanations of many of the symptoms reported above, such as speech sound confusions and reversals, word-finding difficulties, reduced and confused meaning of words, and so on, will be given in terms of disturbed perceptual-linguistic circuitry.

ORAL LANGUAGE DISTURBANCES IN CHILDHOOD

Oral language disturbances may have their origin during the period of audiovocal feedforward and feedback loop development, that is, anything which may interfere with the sequence leading to closed, internal and external audiovocal loops may interfere with later audioverbal development. Problems may also arise, of course, during the sequence leading to closed, internal and external audioverbal loops.

Open, Internal and External Audiovocal Loops. Several factors may keep audiovocal loops from closing at the proper time. For example, there are possibilities of environmental feedforward loop deficits. Environmental feedforward problems may stem from a lack of auditory stimulation, or from a problem in receiving or perceiving such stimulation; such feedforward difficulties may also arise if negative sensations accompany environmental vocalizations.

Figure 6-A illustrates such an open loop. Problems in internal feedback loops may also arise; for example, auditory acuity and perceptual problems may not only interfere with environmental feedforward stimulation but may also interfere with the subject's internal feedback loop or self-stimulation circuit. As an example of where adverse, environmental feed-

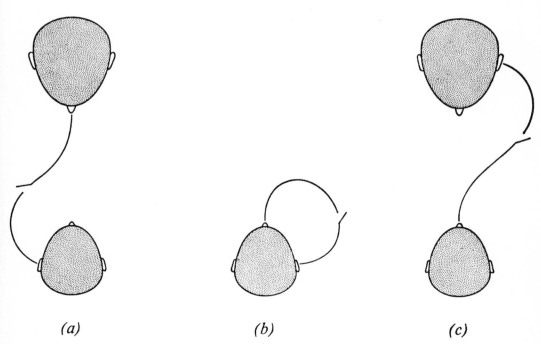

(a)   *(b)*   *(c)*

FIGURE 6. Open audiovocal loops. a. Open, environmental feedforward loop. b. Open, internal feedback loop. c. Open, external feedforward loop.

forward signals eventually disturb subject, internal feedback signals, we may refer back to Mowrer's theory which implies that: if negative sensations are associated with environmental sounds, approximations of these sounds by the child during vocal play may tend to elicit negative sensations within the child and he may eventually reduce his output of these sounds, or he may cease to produce them altogether. Figure 6-B illustrates an open, internal feedback loop. Another situation which may lead to problems in audiovocal loop development is a lack of response from the environment when the child vocalizes to gain attention. Such a lack of environmental response, sometimes planned so as not to "spoil" the child, will tend, if it is rather consistently experienced, to interfere with the development of the child's audiovocal feedforward loop. Figure 6-C shows this type of open loop.

Open, Internal and External Audioverbal Loops. Of course, interference with the closing sequence of audioverbal loop development should also lead to various oral language problems. Specific examples will follow.

Percept Pattern-Heard Word Pattern Loop. In the previous chapter, the significance of perceptual-conceptual development to meaningful oral language development was stressed. It was emphasized that without adequate percept development, heard word and spoken word-pattern developments would be disturbed to varying degrees. This is an important factor to consider here since children with CNS impairment commonly show difficulty in organizing and structuring sensory input and, consequently, may develop distorted and inaccurate percepts. Further, these disturbances are also frequently found in the audiovisual sensory channels.

If such a situation of perceptual dysfunctioning exists, there will be varying degrees of misperception when the child experiences various objects, acts, qualities, or relationships, and hence the heard word-patterns

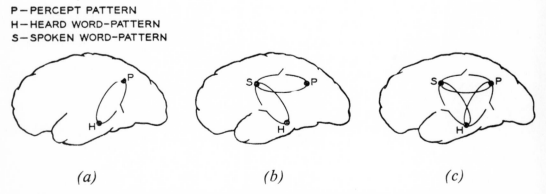

P — PERCEPT PATTERN
H — HEARD WORD-PATTERN
S — SPOKEN WORD-PATTERN

(a)   *(b)*   *(c)*

FIGURE 7. Open audioverbal loops. a. Open, percept pattern-heard word pattern loop. b. Open, percept pattern-spoken word pattern, and open, heard word pattern-spoken word pattern loops. c. Open, internal audioverbal loops.

which accompany these experiences will be less stable and less meaningful. To further complicate the situation, the child, because of auditory perceptual problems, may also be misperceiving the heard word-patterns.

Perceptual conditions, commonly found among brain-damaged children, can be readily seen as interfering with the development of the internal, percept pattern-heard word pattern loop. Figure 7-A shows the left hemisphere and the open loop between important auditory and visual centers of the brain. The figure is presented as a simple illustration of the phenomena discussed.

Reciprocal Relationship Between Percept Pattern and Heard-Word Pattern Loop. Another important step to later speech development is the establishment of an automatic and reciprocal connection between percept pattern and heard word-pattern. That is, if a child perceives an object, or if he should evoke an image of the object, there should be an automatic evocation of the appropriate word or auditory image; and this connection should also become a reciprocal one, so that if the auditory image or heard word-pattern is evoked, there should be an automatic evocation of the appropriate visual image.

It should be evident that if there is difficulty in percept and heard word-pattern development there will also be trouble in the establishment of this very important automatic and reciprocal loop. The latency period of this loop may also be delayed or otherwise disturbed.

Open, Percept Pattern-Spoken Word Pattern Loop, and Open, Heard Word Pattern-Spoken Word Pattern Loop. If there has been difficulty in developing percept patterns and heard word-patterns and automatic and reciprocal relationships between them, there will, of course, be problems in percept pattern—spoken word pattern, and heard word pattern—spoken word pattern activities. These disturbed loops can be detected in many ways. For example, if a child is shown an object and asked for its name, he may not give the appropriate name because he misperceives the object, or he may give a delayed response if the latency period is involved. If there is a problem in the circuit between heard word-patterns and spoken word-patterns, we may observe it during various verbal tasks. For example, the child may give inappropriate responses to yes and no questions or may be unable to respond adequately to word association and analogy tasks. The loop involvements described above are illustrated in Figure 7-B.

Open, Internal Audioverbal Loops. It may be recalled that, if all goes well with audiovocal and audioverbal developmental sequences, the child, at about eighteen months to three years of age, should experience a rapid increase in percept formation. Along with this rapid increase in percept formation is also a concomitant increase in heard word and spoken word-patterns. Important to this discussion is that the child at this time accompanies his perceptual activities with the speech that he is learning; that is, he talks to himself while he perceptualizes. This period may be seen as a time when the child experiences total, internal loop perceptual—linguistic development. In other words, he strengthens the loops between percept patterns, heard word-patterns, and spoken word-patterns by virtue of the fact that as he perceives, he speaks, and listens to what he says.

However, if there have been percept pattern, heard word-pattern or spoken word-pattern loop difficulties, this important self-reporting perceptual-linguistic activity may be disturbed, reduced or absent. Disturbances may also occur, even if proper loop developments have taken place, if adults with mistaken intentions inhibit this activity. Figure 7-C shows this internal, perceptual-linguistic circuitry in the open condition.

Open, External Feedforward and Feedback Audioverbal Loops. Disturbances in external feedforward and feedback audioverbal loops may also occur due to various reasons. The first and obvious reason is based on problems in the closing of previously described feedforward and feedback audiovocal and audioverbal loops. However, specific problems may also stem from: (1) unresponsive listeners, for example, listeners who do not provide regenerative speech feedback, or feedback which indicates the listener is enjoying or appreciative of the speaker's speech attempts; or from unperceived or misperceived positive listener reactions because of the child's perceptual difficulties; and (2) negative environmental feedback arising from listener's who frequently interrupt when the child is having difficulty finding the right word, and from listener's who may overly correct pronunciation or the child's mistaken use of words. The above are examples of degenerative speech feedback and, of course, are very likely to compound the oral linguistic deficits of the child with CNS disturbance.

THERAPY PROCEDURES

Below are suggestions for closing various audiovocal and audioverbal feedforward and feedback loops.

Closing, Pleasure Sensation-Word Production Loop. This discussion on closing the pleasure sensation-word production loop relates to Mowrer's Autism Theory (1958) and his statement that, "if positive emotional connotations can be given to certain sounds, as produced by others, the subject will himself, have a strong disposition to make the responses which produce these sounds." Therefore, if there is a problem in speech maturation, it would be well if the clinician could analyze for whether there are, or whether there were, difficulties experienced in the development of the pleasure sensation-word production loops as illustrated in Figure 5 A-F.

Following are suggestions for helping to close pleasure-word loops, if it is suspected they are deficient. Inspection of Figure 5-A shows that the mature speaker must first provide environmental activities which tend to generate pleasure sensations within the developing speech system. In this regard, the clinician or the parents, should, as often as possible, provide or present interesting play objects, good things to eat, "fun-games" to play, or "fun-places" to go. Before moving to the next step, it should be determined if the therapeutic pleasure activities are, in fact, producing pleasure sensations in the child by observing his facial expressions, and so on. Inspection of Figure 5-B shows that, next, the clinician or parent should accompany these pleasure-producing moments with some word, for example [mɑmɪ], or phrase. If all has gone well to this point, the mature speaker is now providing both environmental, feedforward pleasure sensations and environmental speech signals. Figure 5-C indicates that the steps illustrated in Figures 5-A and B should continue until it becomes apparent that the speaker's speech signal alone elicits good feelings in the child. Again, this fact may be determined by observing the child's facial expressions, body posture and movements when the clinician or parent appears and utters the selected word or phrase. Again, if all has gone well up to this point, it might be expected that when the child engages in random vocalizations, he will elicit good feelings within himself by his approximation of the appropriate word, as illustrated in Figures D and E. In terms of feedback theory, the latter steps may be described as subject-generated, positive feedback signals which tend to cause reverberation or repetition of the speech signal. The last operation, as illustrated in Figure 5-F, involves the clinician's or parent's reinforcing of the newly-acquired word by responding with social-approval behavior such as a smile, a hug, or by praising the child.

It should also be mentioned that if a pleasure-word loop disturbance was found to be a contributory factor in a particular case of an oral language problem, the clinician should counsel the parents against the frequent use of verbal discipline. Similarly, reduced environmental verbalization concomitant with other unpleasant moments experienced by the child might also be suggested. Such activities should contribute toward the goal of closing pleasure sensation-word production loops.

Closing Internal Audioverbal Loops. After the child begins to vocalize or after internal and external audiovocal loops have been closed, possibly as described above, the clinician should turn his attention to techniques for closing first internal, and then external audioverbal loops. Neurophysiologically speaking, this means developing stable neuronal arrangements for percept-patterns, heard word-patterns, and spoken word-patterns.

Percept Patterns. As has previously been stated, meaningful speech depends on well developed percept patterns. The importance of adequate percept-pattern formation to speech development is suggested by the following discussion. An illustration of an open, percept pattern-heard word pattern loop is shown in Figure 7-A; if this loop remains open, or partially open, the percept pattern-spoken word pattern, and the heard word pattern-spoken word pattern loops will also be involved as shown in Figure 7-B, and, consequently, the complete, internal audioverbal circuitry will be involved as illustrated in Figure 7-C. Further, if this condition prevails, it could be stated that the entire oral linguistic circuitry, including both internal and external feedforward and feedback loops, would show deficits. It should be clear then, that speech clinicians have to continue to develop techniques for clarifying, amplifying, integrating, and stabilizing percept patterns. Such techniques are especially important when it is established that a particular speech client suffers from perceptual dysfunctioning. Examples of such techniques follow.

With respect to visual percepts, the clinician could consider the use of oversized objects; he could also make use of color and textural clues as well. In certain cases, associated olfactory and gustatory clues could also be utilized.

To cite a specific example of such percept formation work, let us suppose a clinician is working with a case who shows difficulty in form discrimination. The clinician could certainly begin by using, for example, oversized objects representing roundness and squareness. He could then apply a color cue by making all square objects red and all round objects blue. He could then go further by making all square objects red and rough in texture and all round objects blue and smooth in texture. He could then, if needed, move to even a more primitive sensory channel for association value by applying a certain well defined and distinct scent to the square object and a certain well defined and distinct scent to the round object. These latter procedures would represent an attempt to employ the lower order tactuo-olfactory channels to help in the form discrimination task, and, in effect, this results in a synesthetic or all-sensory channel approach to the problem. It is also suggested that some sort of "natural" order be considered when collecting objects and materials to be used in percept formation therapy. For example, the clinician should begin with the perceptual-field point of reference, that is, the self (body parts), and then he should move outwards to family members, food, clothing, home (e.g., rooms, furniture), and, finally, out into the surrounding environment (trees, plants, vehicles, animals, etc.).

Heard Word-patterns. In the case of heard word-patterns, the clinician could help to integrate and strengthen them by the use of amplification; by manipulating loudness, pitch, quality, and duration factors; and by manipulating the factor of background sound. Various combinations of such heard word-pattern manipulation must be tried in order to discover which combination is best for any particular client. Following percept-pattern work, then, there should be concentration on heard word-pattern work; this rather self-evident statement is made here because so often children who are having difficulty in developing speech are often asked and cajoled by adults in the environment to produce utterances. It would be much more efficient, if instead, those who wished to help would concentrate on developing percept and heard word-patterns, and, thereby, hopefully allowing spoken word-patterns to emerge more or less spontaneously.

As with percept-pattern work, the clinician should consider various techniques to facilitate the development of heard word-patterns. Following are some suggestions.

Since children first learn to react to gestures (Latif, 1934), and also first understand "body English" (postures, expressions) and tonal aspects of vocalization before they comprehend heard-word patterns, the clinician could make good use of these association-value factors in his heard word-pattern therapy program. For example, the clinician could use gestures alone or gestures plus words while engaging the child in various "give me," "point to," "get me," "show me" verbal games. Periodically, the "body English" could be reduced in order to determine how well heard word-patterns may be developing.

Spoken Word-patterns. Theoretically, spoken word-patterns follow rather spontaneously the establishment of percept and heard word-patterns. However, when specific attempts at eliciting vocalization become necessary, the following developmental sequence should be kept in mind.

It could be supported that random or unorganized vocalization and random or unorganized bodily activity represent the initial stage in the development of spoken word-patterns. Following this unorganized body and vocal activity, is the stage marked by the organization of bodily activity into body language (i.e., meaningful gesture, pantomime, facial expressions, body postures) plus random vocalization. Then follows the development of body language in association with the initial organization of vocalization (i.e., lower order onomatopoesis such as gr-r-r-r, z-z-z, or ba-a-a-a for animal sounds, or higher order onomatopoesis such as bang, splash, click, pop, snap, etc.) and, finally, body language in association with organized vocalization.

Loop-closing Techniques. Specific techniques for closing percept pattern-heard word pattern loops include:

1. Imagery feedback activities. The clinician presents an object and asks the child to "study" it. Then, the clinician asks the child to close his eyes and to see the object in his mind's eye, so to speak. The child may be asked to examine the object again and to attend to textural sensations, or to taste and smell sensations whenever appropriate. Again, the child may be requested to experience the sensations with his mind's fingers, nose, or mouth. Next, the clinician utters the appropriate spoken word-pattern which represents the object and asks the child to "listen" once again for the word but this time with his mind's ear. Finally, the child may be asked to "listen" to the word and then to "see" the object; to "listen" to the word and then to "feel" the object; to "listen" to the word and then to "smell" the object, and so on. These activities should contribute to various types of perceptual-imagery looping.

2. *Intraverbalizing activities.* Following work on closing, percept pattern-heard word pattern loops, attempts should be aimed at integrating the internal, spoken word-pattern loop with percept and heard word-patterns. Such techniques have been described in a recent article by the present writer (Mysak, 1961) and similar ones by Van Riper (1963, Ch. 14). The techniques involve clinician intraverbalizing or self-reporting of certain activities, as well as oral reporting by the clinician of the client's activities. Both of these verbal activities are done with the hope of eventually initiating intraverbalizing behavior on the part of the client, and thus serving the purpose of integrating the spoken word-pattern loop with percept and heard word-patterns.

For example, the clinician may speak aloud in a simple fashion, that is, by using appropriate single words, or phrases, while manipulating human figures and furniture in the presence of the child. Or, he may produce appropriate speech units while the child manipulates such objects. It should be noted that body language could be employed as accompaniment to the monologues in instances where body language is needed to support the speech units.

Closing External Audioverbal Loops. Successful closing of internal audioverbal loops should eventually result in an increased amount of interverbalizing. However, specific attention may be given to closing external audioverbal loops by making use of the following techniques.

Auditory Closure Activities. The clinician may employ the technique of auditory closure of speech units as one way of helping to close external audioverbal loops. For example, he may present a series of incomplete statements such as, "When I am tired, I go to _____;" "When I am hungry, I _____;" "I live in a _____." Such incomplete statements can be organized into categories and made more difficult as work progresses; further, a steadily increasing number of words can be omitted. The exercise could include the completion of story units begun by the clinician as well.

Additional techniques here may be based on test items from a recently described test of psycholinguistic abilities (Kirk and McCarthy, 1961).

For example, the child may be asked to answer "yes" or "no," to questions such as "Do birds fly?;" he may be asked to respond to analogies such as "Birds sing, dogs _____;" and he may be shown a series of objects and asked "to tell" about them.

Definitions, Antonyms and Synonyms. During the verbal game of definitions, the child may be asked to define a word, or may be given a definition and asked for the best word; whereas, in the antonym-synonym verbal exercise, the child is asked simply to provide similar or opposite words to various stimulus words.

Dialogue Improvisation. Dialogue improvisation is done by first having the clinician re-create a meaningful situation—such as with mother or with father, at school, at the store, at the zoo, and so on—by the use of appropriate props. Then the clinician should begin the dialogue and encourage the child to join in.

Buildup and Breakdown. The verbal exercise of "buildup" and "breakdown" is engaged in by presenting a word, for example, "horse" and requesting the child to analyze the idea of the word, that is, the child should respond by saying, head, tail, hoof, and so on; and then by requesting the child to elaborate on the idea of the word, that is, the child should respond by saying, dog, cat, sheep, and so on.

Look-do-speak. The look-do-speak verbal activity is done by first collecting large, simple action pictures, for example, a boy batting a ball, a man striking a nail, a girl chasing a dog, a child opening a present, and so on. The clinician indicates what should be done by turning the first picture face up and responding to the picture with appropriate action, body language, and speech units.

Auditory Memory Span, Analysis, and Synthesis. Sharpening auditory perceptual functioning may be done by having the child repeat progressively longer words, phrases, and sentences; and also by having the child reduce certain words into their component syllables, or to synthesize words from their component syllables.

Verbal Associations. In the verbal association exercise, the client is encouraged to utter the first words that are evoked by various stimulus words.

Loop Latency Period. During attempts at the above-described techniques, consideration should be given to the integration-response latency period. In other words, the clinician should allow more than the usual amount of time for the child to associate percept with heard word-patterns, or heard word-patterns with appropriate speech units. For example, having the child repeat the first part of the incomplete statement, or having the child repeat the question might be helpful because it allows the child a longer integration-response latency period.

Redundancy and Restructuring. When directing speech signals at a client who may be experiencing comprehension difficulty, the clinician should make sure to attempt to repeat the message, to overstate it, to simplify the syntax, and so on, before abandoning the attempted communication.

Verbal Assists. During attempts at oral communication, the clinician should use freely the following verbal supports: representative objects and pictures, body language, and onomatopoesis.

Additional "Logocybernetic" Techniques. Before concluding the section on therapy procedures, an elaboration of certain techniques described in Chapter Two will be presented.

Regenerative Speech Feedback. It may be recalled again that regenerative speech feedback is that which comes from a listener and which indicates to the speaker that the listener is interested in and enjoying what is being said. It has been stated that such external loop signals will very often cause an increase in the speaker's output, and hence speech clinicians, involved with language-disturbed clients, should learn how best to generate such feedforward signals. For instance, much in the way of regenerative speech signals may be reflected by the clinician's assuming certain facial expressions at the appropriate time during the client's speech attempts, or by inserting appropriate 'feeder' words or phrases such as, "really," "no kidding," and "tell me more."

Double, Multiple Speech Feedback. As previously stated, multiple speech feedback refers to that process whereby speech is monitored by more than one sensory channel, for example, by various combinations of auditory, tactile, and proprioceptive channels. Double, multiple speech feedback is experienced when a listener attends closely to a speaker, anticipates certain words because of a familiarity with what is about to be said, and speaks simultaneously (fraction of a second lag between the lead speaker and the follower) in slave fashion with the lead speaker. The listener, thereby, receives double auditory, tactile, and proprioceptive feedbacks associated with the speaker's utterances. Echo speaking, where the listener repeats words or phrases after the speaker, may be regarded as delayed, multiple speech feedback. The stimulation of such slave or echo speech may be found useful when attempting to specifically initiate external, audioverbal feedforward signals from the client.

Related to these ideas are the findings of a recent study (Copeland, 1963) of the effects of feedback modification on the verbal behavior of retardates. The investigator was interested in the possible use of modified feedback as a facilitator of speech output. In short, the child's own vocalizations were fed back to him in a solitary situation after a certain specified delay time. A similar opportunity for vocalization was offered without the feedback condition. One of the findings of the study was that the feedback condition elicited a significantly greater amount of vocalization than did the non-feedback condition.

Alloplastic and Autoplastic Speech Characteristics. It was stated in Chapter Two that an alloplastic speech system is one which depends on the conversational partner to initiate or maintain a conversation, while an autoplastic speech system assumes the initiative and carries the conversation. It was also mentioned that an ideal speech system would possess a proper balance of both alloplastic and autoplastic features.

In therapy for language-involved children, the speech clinician should seek ways to stimulate the autoplastic features of the child's oral linguistic circuitry. Some of the ways in which this might be done are: (1) by stimulating certain emotional states which tend to facilitate verbalization, for example, by presenting objects which the child may want to explore and then withholding them until the child attempts utterances, or by bringing the child into stimulating environments such as an airport, subway, fire station, zoo, and so on; (2) by initiating speech behavior and then pretending to need help in finding words or completing thoughts; and (3) by indicating to the child that he is especially good in explaining certain ideas, and so on.

FEEDBACK DISTURBANCES IN APHASIA

Before concluding this chapter, it might be instructive to connect some of the expressed feedback concepts with certain problems of, and therapy procedures for, adults who suffer from aphasia.

Aphasic Problems. Aphasia indicates the presence of oral linguistic entropy, that is, the presence of a disorder which increases oral linguistic confusion and decreases oral linguistic order. The basic disorder causing the aphasia may be responsible for opening, for example, the percept pattern-heard word pattern loop, or the heard word pattern-spoken word pattern loop, or the percept pattern-spoken word pattern loop—or, in other words, to various degrees and combinations, the client's internal, and external, audioverbal feedforward and feedback loops. Such disturbances may, of course, affect conceptual activity as well.

Additionally, in terms of the ten operations involved in a full speech cycle as described in Chapter Two, the aphasic may not only suffer from the more commonly recognized oral language symptoms, but may also suffer from deficits in thought pattern-word pattern comparing (inner speech monitoring); word product-thought pattern comparing (actual speech monitoring); and word product-listener reaction comparing (awareness of error speech based on evaluating listener reactions). Further, changes in audioverbal loop latency periods accompanying cases of aphasia may also be overlooked by clinicians. That is, aphasics may need more time to engage mechanisms responsible for the automatic and reciprocal connections between heard word-patterns and percept patterns, or between percept patterns and spoken word-patterns; and this condition may be aggravated by the tendency for many aphasics to attempt to utilize their premorbid integration-formulation-transmission latency periods (in some cases, this tendency may turn out to be the major problem). Eventually, unsuccessful speech efforts, on the part of aphasics with latency period lags, engender secondary language problems which complicate the symptomatology.

Therapy Techniques. Following are a few examples of anti-entropic oral language therapy techniques.

Off-setting Latency Period Lags. To counteract latency period disturbances in various audioverbal loops, the client may be asked, for example, not to respond to a question until he has formulated his response in his mind and scanned it for content. Or, on the integration side, the client may be asked to refrain from answering a question until he has repeated the question aloud as well as silently in his mind. These techniques often bring results and may confirm the clinician's suspicion that an important part of a particular aphasic's problem is related to latency period lags in various parts of his oral linguistic circuitry.

Body Language Support. It may be recalled that body language development precedes oral language development, and that eventually organized body language accompanies oral language. However, as the individual matures, he may use less and less accompanying body language to support his oral language since his oral language becomes increasingly more efficient as a function of maturation. The clinician may find however that if a particular aphasic, who exhibits difficulty in transmitting speech signals, were to lead his oral attempts with appropriate body language, his efforts at oral language might be facilitated. In this instance, the clinician, by utilizing such a technique, is contributing to his client's language rehabilitation by re-activating the primitive loop between his client's body and oral languages. Again, on the integration side, the clinician may discover that, when communicating with his client, he may facilitate his client's integration processes by supporting his oral language with generous amounts of body language.

Internal Loop Feedback. Under the therapy category of closing internal feedback loops, the client may be asked a question, asked to formulate a potential response, and then asked to intentionally scan the potential response for any error factors before transmitting it. The client may also be asked to formulate more than one possible response, to scan as many as he can hold in mind, to select the shortest and the clearest, and then to transmit it.

Further, as he transmits his response, he may be asked to intentionally over-monitor his word production and to comment on how it might have been further refined. As an assist here, the clinician could amplify the client's speech feedback.

External Loop Feedback. To assist in closing external feedback loops in those cases where it is necessary, the client may be asked to intentionally scan listener reactions for expected or desired responses, then to form opinions about the listener reactions, and, finally, to compare these opinions with actual listener reactions by questioning the listener.

SUMMARY

1. Certain literature on language disorders in children is reviewed and

the problems discussed are placed under categories of disorders in audition, words and word arrangement, and word meanings.

2. Oral language disturbances in children are presented in terms of open, internal and external audiovocal loops, and open, internal and external audioverbal loops. Factors which may contribute to audiovocal loop disturbances are: environmental feedforward deficits based on reduced stimulation, or acuity, or perceptual dysfunctioning; negative emotional sensations accompanying environmental vocalization, and reduced environmental response to the child's vocalizations. Factors which may contribute to audioverbal loop disturbances are: open, percept pattern-heard word pattern; open, percept pattern-spoken word pattern; and open, heard word pattern-spoken word pattern loops.

3. Therapy procedures for children are presented and include techniques for closing the pleasure sensation-word production loop; closing internal audioverbal loops (e.g., attention given to percept patterns, heard word-patterns, spoken word-patterns, imagery feedback, and intraverbalizing activities); and closing external audioverbal loops (e.g., auditory closure activities, as well as work on definitions, look-do-speak activity, work on verbal buildup-breakdown exercises, verbal associations, etc.).

4. Certain additional logocybernetic therapy techniques are also presented and are based on: regenerative speech feedback techniques; double, multiple-speech feedback technique; and techniques associated with stimulating autoplastic speech characteristics.

5. Certain relatively neglected symptoms of aphasia are also briefly discussed. These include problems of thought pattern-word pattern comparing; word product-thought pattern comparing; word product-listener reaction comparing; and lags in audioverbal loop latency periods. Counteracting therapy techniques are presented such as: off-setting latency period lags, body language support, and techniques for closing internal and external audioverbal loops.

REFERENCES

COPELAND, R. H.: 2. The effects of feedback modification on verbal behavior. *J. Speech Hearing Dis. (Monogr.), 10:*70-75, 1963.

HAGBERG, B.: The sequelae of spontaneously arrested infantile hydrocephalus. *Develop. Med. Child Neurol., 4:*583-587, 1962.

INGRAM, T. T. S.: Pediatric aspects of specific developmental dysphasia, dyslexia, and dysgraphia. *Cereb. Palsy Bull., 2:*254-277, 1960.

KIRK, S. A., and McCARTHY, J. J.: The Illinois test of psycholinguistic abilities—an approach to differential diagnosis. *Amer. J. Ment. Defic., 66:*399-412, 1961.

LATIF, I.: The physiological basis of linguistic development and of the ontogeny of meaning: I, II. *Psychol. Rev., 41:*55-85, 153-176, 1934.

LEWIS, R. S., STRAUSS, A. A., and LEHTINEN, LAURA, E.: *The Other Child.* New York, Grune and Stratton, 1960.

Mowrer, O. H.: Hearing and speaking: an analysis of language learning. *J. Speech Hearing Dis.*, 23:143-152, 1958.

Mysak, E. D.: Organismic development of oral language. *J. Speech Hearing Dis.*, 26:377-384, 1961.

Strauss, A. A., and Kephart, N. C.: *Psychopathology and Education of the Brain-Injured Child, Vol. 2.* New York, Grune and Stratton, 1955.

Van Riper, C.: *Speech Correction 4th Ed.* Englewood Cliffs, Prentice-Hall, 1963.

Chapter Five

TONAL GENERATION

In this chapter, voicing or tonal generation will be discussed primarily in terms of its control and its rehabilitation.

For good reviews of the literature on voice disorders and voice rehabilitation, the reader is referred to *Voice and Articulation* (Van Riper and Irwin, Ch. 7-9), the *Handbook of Speech Pathology* (1957, Ch. 22, 26), *Vocal Rehabilitation* (Brodnitz, 1959) and the large work *Voice-Speech-Language* (Luchsinger and Arnold, 1965, pp. 167-334). Further, the present author, within a chapter entitled, "Phonatory and Resonatory Problems" (Mysak, 1966), presented a review of recent literature on vocal evolution and involution, the concept of normal and abnormal voicing, laryngeal correlates of vocal attributes, and voice disorders of infraglottal, glottal, and supraglottal origins.

The specific goal of this chapter is to discuss the critical factor of audioregulation of phonation and to present therapy techniques based on this discussion.

PHONOCYBERNETIC THEORY

In Chapter One, certain studies were reported (i.e., Black, 1959, Hanley and Draegart, 1949) which supported the concept that the ear has the property of a voice control system and, therefore, is an important mechanism for adjusting phonatory behavior. Interesting and pertinent findings of two additional investigators will be reviewed now, in order to further justify the cybernation of vocal behavior in this chapter.

Stromsta (1959) indicates that it appears supportable to state ". . . that phonation as well as speech perse is affected or controlled by audition concurrent to the activity." He states further that:

> If the "control signal" can be assumed to be a composite of bone-tissue and air-conduction sidetone transduced to the central nervous system then facts related to the pathways of sidetone would tend to indicate that the composite signal is possibly an aberration of the actual acoustic event. If this be the case, the extent of aberration inherent in the normal speaker in a conventional acoustic environment speculatively must fall within the limiting conditions of the auditory control system whereas certain experimentally induced aberrations would be seen as exceeding the limits of the control system as shown by quantifiable variations. In like manner, it is

[63]

tempting to think that certain difficulties of speech are due to inherent aberration that exceeds the limits of the control system.

One aim of the study conducted by Stromsta was to determine the effects of air-conduction sidetone signal distortion on the phonation of a sustained vowel. He found that sidetone signal distortion resulted in the blockage of phonation, in extreme pitch variations, and in undersirable voice quality.

On the basis of Stromsta's work, it is conceivable that some voice problems may be due to certain differences in auditory systems which prevent these auditory systems from using efficiently their voice control function. Further, this suggests that successful voice therapy in these instances would depend upon certain therapeutic intrusions into, or modifications of, the individual's auditory feedback.

Tomatis (1963, Ch. 4) offers some interesting ideas concerning audition, phonation, and cybernetics in a chapter entitled, "Audio-Phonology." He, too, is convinced that the ear receives, regulates, and pilots phonation, and that the voice, its inflections and its timbre depends on this auditory control function. In support of his statements, Tomatis refers to a series of experiments which he conducted with professional singers. He describes one instance where he induced auditory fatigue with high level noise and then observed the complete loss of vocal control within the singer. The singer's vocal control returned as the effects of the auditory fatigue wore off. Tomatis also reported on the effects on singer's voices when certain frequencies were filtered out of their auditory feedbacks. For example, when frequencies above 2,000 cps were filtered out, there was a quality change and the voice became dull and toneless. In short, Tomatis believes a subject is capable of phonating only what he can control auditorially.

The controversial topic of the dominant ear is discussed by Tomatis in another chapter of his book (1963, Ch. 6). He describes an experiment in which he had an individual sing into an apparatus which allowed the experimenter to feed back the subject's voice into both ears of the singer, or into either his left or right ear. It was found that during bilateral and right unilateral auditory stimulation, no adverse effects on singing were noted; however, when the voice was fed back into the singer's left ear only, the singer's voice lost all its professional qualities. Similarly, when an actor's speech was fed back into his left ear only, his voice lost its timbre. Tomatis is convinced that a dominant ear exists for regulating the singing as well as the speaking voice.

Again, the above findings emphasize the importance of audioregulation of phonation. The findings also suggest that clinicians might find it interesting to investigate whether, in any one of their particular clients, something like a dominant ear for audiovocal control is operative; and whether therapy techniques, based on the concept of a preferred ear, have anything to offer such a client.

AUDIOREGULATION IN VOICE THERAPY

There have been at least two attempts to outline voice therapy based on feedback ideas. Van Riper and Irwin (1958, pp. 284-288) describe a plan which includes techniques for identifying a more suitable voice pattern; scanning for the purpose of comparing a desired voice pattern with the actual voice, and making attempts to modify the voice in the direction of the desired pattern; and, finally, techniques for fixing and stabilizing the new voice. Shearer (1959) has also presented a short cybernetically-oriented outline for voice therapy. Briefly, he suggests laryngeal muscle exercises to increase the client's vocal flexibility, and techniques designed to cause the client to "forget" his habitual voice pattern and to begin seeking for a new and more appropriate one.

With the preceding comments serving as introduction, the remaining sections of the chapter will be devoted to an outline of audioregulation and voice therapy.

Reverse Tonal-symbol, Figure-ground Relationship. As the initial step in voice therapy, attention should be paid to reversing the figure-ground relationship between the spoken symbol and the carrier tone which conveys the symbol. This means developing techniques which will cause the client to re-experience, in effect, his infantile, audiovocal loop feedforward-feedback developmental sequence. To state the idea in another way, the clinician should devise ways of getting his client to monitor primarily his voicing, rather than to monitor primarily his speech content. Further, monitoring of vocalization should be done on an intentional or "thinking brain" level rather than on the usual nonintentional or "doing brain" level.

Before discussing techniques for reversing the tonal-symbol, figure-ground relationship, it would serve the purpose of this portion of the chapter to present a brief review of how an individual originally identifies and establishes his voice pattern by referring back to the discussion on the development of audiovocal and audioverbal loops as found in Chapter Three. During the first year, or the audiovocal loop development period, the sequence includes: (1) an early period of response to the environmental human voice by cessation of, for example, whimpering (initiation of the incorporation of a parental model tone), and unorganized and apparently unmonitored voicing such as crying and screaming; (2) a smile response to the mother's voice (continuation of the incorporation of the parental model tone), and the production of more organized intonations along with a growing response to these self-produced sounds as shown, for example, by personal facial expressions; (3) motor responses to the calling of his name (further model tone incorporation, and a transition from just responding to tonal, to tonal plus symbol stimulation), and the continuing production of organized intonations, but now with a tendency to repeat self-produced sounds (establishment of infantile audioregulation of vocal output); and (4) an increased awareness and comprehension of tonal symbols, and an increased tendency toward not only repetition of self-produced sounds but also repetition of environmental model sounds. It may be recalled that a similar sequence is observed during audioverbal loop development, that is, first there is primarily self-talking, then there is more and more listening to environmental symbols, and, finally, there is more and more talking to others.

The important points to remember for purposes of our present discussion are: (1) the progressive incorporation by the individual of a model voice pattern; (2) the sequence of apparently no auditory regulation of vocal output, to a progressively greater amount, and, finally, to an established audioregulation; and (3) the sequence of attending first to tonal, and then to tonal plus symbol aspects of environmental voicing, and the sequence of monitoring first just tonal, and then tonal plus symbol aspects of self-produced vocalization. It is believed the client will tend to persist in the use of his habitual, inefficient voice pattern unless the clinician can get the client to begin listening once again to environmental tones rather than primarily symbols; and can get the client to begin listening once again to his own tones rather than primarily his own symbols. Suggested techniques for reversing the tonal-symbol, figure-ground relationship follow.

The important first step on the part of the client for re-experiencing audiovocal loop monitoring is for him to be able to "de-symbolize" his vocalization, so that tonal generation may again emerge as the auditory figure rather than as the auditory background. Toward this purpose, the clinician may prepare lists of nonsense words, phrases, sentences and story units for the client to vocalize. At this stage, the client is asked merely to vocalize and that is all. This corresponds with the first stage of audiovocal loop development. Here, it might be well to remind the clinician of the need to fully explain to the client the reason for attempting to reverse the tonal-symbol, figure-ground relationship, so as to ensure the client's fullest cooperation in performing the assigned task. After the client is able to vocalize nonsense material easily and well and has done so on a daily basis, as well as during therapy sessions, the second stage of work may be begun. The only addition in the second stage is that the client is now requested to intentionally listen to his own vocalization. Now the client's nonsense vocalization may also be recorded and played back for his scrutiny. He may also vocalize into an amplification system. Or, the clinician may imitate the client's faulty voice pattern and ask the client to study the pattern. Once the client has "saturated" his ears with his own error-voice pattern and can describe all its dimensions well, the clinician may move on to the third stage of therapy. In the third stage, the clinician should add to his lists, practice material loaded with reduplicative nonsense words, phrases, sentences, and story units. Now the client is asked to vocalize and to assume a self-listening attitude each time a reduplicative sound pattern appears and to repeat the unit once or twice. This corresponds with the stage of audio-vocal loop development where the child repeats self-produced sounds. Exercises based on simulating conversation with nonsense speech units might also be used as a supplementary exercise here.

It is hoped that after such activity at least three things have occurred: (1) that the client is listening once again to tonal as well as symbol aspects of his phonatory behavior; (2) that there has been some change in the tonal-symbol, figure-ground relationship; and (3) that the client has developed a keen appreciation of the pitch, intensity, quality, and durational dimensions of his error-voice pattern.

Error-voice Sensitivity and Error-voice Measuring. The next phase in therapy involves the development within the client of sensitivity to any pitch, intensity, quality, and durational error dimensions of his voicing, and to stimulate the client toward recognizing the type and extent of these error factors. In terms of the functions and components of the cybernetic analogue of the speech system, the clinician plans: (1) to disrupt the predicted zero error signal for voicing which exists within the client's product comparator; (2) to cause the client's comparator to begin measuring and determining the error factors contained in the client's vocal output; and (3) to trigger the client's voice corrector device. At least three therapy steps may be taken in order to activate client error-sensitivity and error-measuring.

Locating A More Efficient Voice Pattern. First, the client, with the aid of the previously prepared nonsense material (used to maintain the therapeutically appropriate tonal-symbol, figure-ground relationship), is asked to vocalize the material in as many different ways as he can. For example, he may vocalize and intentionally modify first the pitch dimension; then the intensity dimension; then the quality dimension; and, finally, the durational dimension of his phonatory pattern. This activity should be continued until the client has substantially increased his ability to modify the various dimensions of his voice, and until the clinician has recognized a voice pattern produced by the client which appears to be a suitable replacement for the client's error pattern. The clinician may find it advantageous if he does some "vocal leading" of the client toward more efficient voice patterns. Much of this vocalization can be recorded, and analyzed by both the client and the clinician for signs of increased ability on the part of the client to vary the different dimensions of voice, and for voice patterns which sound better. In time, the client and clinician should agree on the most suitable pattern, or the one which gives the most voice for the least amount of effort.

Once this pattern has been identified, the client may be asked to record samples of nonsense words, phrases, and conversational units using the new voice, for use in later stages of therapy.

Establishing the Correct-voice Pattern. Once the more efficient voice pattern has been identified and samples recorded, the client is again required to re-experience the audiovocal loop developmental sequence, but this time using the more efficient voice pattern. Again, the client merely vocalizes the nonsense material with the more efficient voice pattern, then vocalizes the material while intentionally listening to it. Here again these attempts may be recorded and scrutinized and vocalized under amplification. Finally, the client vocalizes the material loaded with reduplicatives and again repeats the reduplicatives once or twice, and so on. Following this activity, it is hoped that the client's listening to tonal rather than symbol aspects of voicing has been reinforced and that the client has developed a keen appreciation of all the dimensions of the correct-voice pattern.

Comparing Error-voice and Correct-voice Patterns. Identification and measuring of error factors is again done with tonal rather than symbol material. Nonsense phrases can be read first with the error pattern and then with the correct pattern, recorded, and error factors analyzed and discussed. The client and clinician could also vocalize simultaneously—first the client may use the error voice and the clinician the correct voice, and vice versa. During these activities, the client may be asked again to identify error factors in his voice.

It should be useful here to describe an instrument which was constructed for use by the Teachers College Speech and Hearing Center. It is an instrument which contains a monitoring set of earphones with a microphone for the client, and a monitoring set of earphones with a microphone for the clinician. The clinician possesses controls which allow him the following voice transmission modes: (1) bilateral self-stimulation of the client; (2) right or left ear unilateral self-stimulation of the client; and (3) right ear self-stimulation by the client, and simultaneous left ear stimulation from the clinician, and vice versa, and a "fader" control which allows the clinician to gradually attenuate the client's voice, while the clinician's voice is gradually amplified, or vice versa.

With this type of apparatus, many of the techniques described above can be carried out more easily. For example, under the heading, comparing error-voice and correct-voice patterns, the clinician could adjust the instrument so that he feeds the client's error voice first into one ear and then into the other; or he feeds the client's error voice into one ear and the correct voice into the other, or reverses the process; or the error voice could be fed into the client's right ear, while simultaneously, the clinician stimulates the client's left ear with the correct voice, and so on. Another interesting possibility is fading out the error voice while simultaneously amplifying the correct voice. It has been found that under such a situation the individual whose personal voice feedback is gradually being attenuated will modify his voice in the direction of the amplified, model phonatory pattern. That is, if the client is producing the error voice and his voice is being fed back into his left ear, and the clinician is simultaneously producing the correct voice and is feeding this voice into the client's right ear, and the clinician gradually attenuates the client's voice feedback while amplifying his own voice, the client's voice may be observed to modify in the direction of the clinician's voice. In other words, vocal homeostasis is disturbed when the client is producing one type of vocal pattern while hearing a different one. This homeostasis can be re-established if the client adjusts his voice to match that which he is hearing.

Correct-voice Seeking and Approximating. If there has been successful adjustment of the tonal-symbol, figure-ground relationship, and activation of error-voice sensitivity and error-voice measuring, the speech system should no longer automatically process the error voice as a carrier for spoken symbols and the speech product corrector (vocal aspect) should become operative. Under this situation, the client should find that, somewhere along in the therapy program, his speaking attempts will be associated with vocal seeking for, and approximating of, the correct voice pattern.

Re-establishment of Appropriate Tonal-symbol, Figure-ground Relationship. As the process of error-voice sensitivity, error measuring, seeking, and approximating proceeds successfully, there will be a gradual re-establishment of the pre-therapy tonal-symbol, figure-ground relationship. In other words, after a new and efficient voice pattern is established, this pattern will be monitored via a "ground" monitoring system, while the symbol will again be monitored via a "figure" monitoring system.

ADDITIONAL PHONOCYBERNETIC THERAPY TECHNIQUES

Following are a few additional feedback therapy procedures.

Imagery Voice Feedback. The individual may be asked to practice his new voice under the regulation of his mind's ear as often as possible during the day. This should contribute to sharpening product comparator and corrector functions.

Unilateral Voice Feedback (after Tomatis). It may be found that therapy progress is facilitated by either masking one ear or the other, or by allowing voice feedback into only one ear or the other. In most cases, the right ear should give the best results.

Alteration of Auditory Feedback. Tomatis (1963, Ch. 4) describes the use of an instrument whereby a singer receives his voice back, but his audition has been electronically altered so that his hearing has been "enriched." Under these circumstances, his vocalization responds in accordance with his altered audition. (The reader may have experienced something akin to enriched feedback while singing or speaking in the shower, or in a room with unusual reverberation characteristics and, consequently, had his voice react accordingly.) This is similar in a way to the "fading" procedure previously described where the client's hearing is "enriched" by the clinician's voice, while the client's voice feedback is gradually eliminated.

SUMMARY

1. The concept of audioregulation of voice control is supported by referring to studies by Black, Hanley and Draegart, Stromsta, and Tomatis. Further, it is stated that many voice problems may be based on deficits in the auditory control system.

2. Audioregulatory voice therapy is described and includes techniques designed to reverse the tonal-symbol, figure-ground relationship, and activate error-voice sensitivity and measuring and correct-voice seeking and approximating.

3. Additional phonocybernetic therapy techniques such as imagery voice feedback, unilateral voice feedback, and auditory feedback modification are also described.

REFERENCES

BLACK, J. W.: The loudness of sidetone. *Speech Monogr.*, *21*:301-305, 1954.

BRODNITZ, F .S.: *Vocal Rehabilitation*. Minnesota: Whiting Press, 1959.

HANLEY, T. D., and DRAEGART, G. L.: Effect of level of distracting noise upon speaking rate, duration, and intensity. Tech. Rept. SCD 104-2-14, Contract N6 or 1-104, T.C. 11, 1949.

LUCHSINGER, R., and ARNOLD, G. E.: *Voice-Speech-Language*. Belmont, Wadsworth, 1965.

MYSAK, E. D.: Phonatory and resonatory problems. In: *Speech Pathology*, R. W. Rieber, and R. S. Brubaker, Ed. Amsterdam, North-Holland Publishing, 1966.

SHEARER, W. M.: Cybernetics in the treatment of voice disorders. *J. Speech Hearing Dis.*, 24:280-282, 1959.

STROMSTA, C.: Experimental blockage of phonation by distorted sidetone. *J. Speech Hearing Res.*, 2:286-301, 1959.

TOMATIS, A.: *L'oreille et le Language*. Paris, Editions du Seuil, 1963.

TRAVIS, L. E., Ed.:*Handbook of Speech Pathology*. New York, Appleton, 1957.

VAN RIPER, C., and IRWIN, J. W.: *Voice and Articulation*. Englewood Cliffs, Prentice-Hall, 1958.

Chapter Six

TONAL MODULATION

Tonal modulation, or the stopping or constricting of an intoned or non-intoned breathstream by action of the articulatory system for the purpose of producing the sound units of speech, is the subject of this chapter.

The chapter will be divided into sections devoted to the normal acquisition of speech sounds, to abnormal speech sound acquisition, and, finally, to remedial procedures.

NORMAL ACQUISITION OF SPEECH SOUNDS

It should be noted that some of the terms used here in describing speech sound acquisition have been used in similar ways by other authors. The terms scanning and comparing, for example, have been used by Van Riper and Irwin (1958, Ch. 6), and the term word approximation has been used by McCurry and Irwin (1953).

Auditory Orienting. The infant's major sensory channel for speech sound reception, perception, and control is the auditory channel. Hence, one of the first phases in speech sound acquisition is marked by the orienting of the infant toward the source of human vocalization. As was described in Chapter Three, the auditory orientation sequence is as follows: auditory startle (e.g., body stiffening, eye blinking, crying) in response to an unexpected loud sound; auditory staring (immobilization of the eyes) in response to certain sounds; auditory searching (side-to-side head movements) in response to sound; and, finally, auditory localizing, or the turning of the head and eyes towards the source of sound. Auditory localization behavior, such as the ability to localize the mother's voice, is established by six months of age. Auditory orientation toward the source of human sound, then, is considered to be a first and necessary step toward the acquisition of speech sounds.

Auditory Scanning. In Chapter Two, scanning was described as that process whereby a mechanism explores and selectively brings to attention those items which are appropriate for a particular problem situation. If the problem situation is the careful examination of speech sounds, external loop, speech-sound scanning would describe the careful scrutiny by a listener of speech sounds being uttered by a speaker, whereas internal loop, speech-sound scanning would describe the careful self-scrutiny by a speaker of his own speech sound production.

[71]

Therefore, after the child has oriented toward the source of sound, an important second phase in speech sound acquisition is the activation of the child's speech-sound auditory scanner. That is, it is necessary for the child to be able to scrutinize the various speech sounds being heard and to bring to his own attention their distinguishing features.

Auditory Tracking. Auditory tracking describes the third phase in speech sound acquisition. In this instance, the child, after orienting toward and scanning for certain speech sounds as produced by another, attempts to produce auditory events which tend to duplicate those which he has heard.

Such tracking attempts may take place immediately after the sounds have been produced by a speaker, namely, by echoic tracking; or, they may take place almost simultaneously with the speaker, namely, by slave tracking. Further, if the sound under scrutiny has been heard often enough by the child, he may develop an auditory image of the sound pattern, and hence he may be able to experience or to evoke the sound pattern in his mind. Attempts at tracking such auditory images of speech sounds may be referred to as imagery tracking.

Auditory Comparing. Speech sound comparing describes a process whereby the child hears the model sound, attempts to reproduce it, and then compares his idea of the intended sound with the product of his actual attempt at sound reproduction. Comparing can take place after the model sound has been produced or during the time it is being produced. In either case, for true comparing to occur, there should be some auditory persistence, or after-hearing of the model sound, so that the child can better compare his sound with the model sound. Problems in developing after-sounds, or in developing after-sounds of adequate duration, may affect the comparing process, and hence interfere with the accurate acquisition of certain speech sounds.

Auditory Approximating. Auditory approximating describes that process whereby the child scans, tracks, and compares speech sounds, and where he may become aware of error signals associated with the comparison between desired and actual speech sound reproduction, and, consequently, where he attempts to track again. In short, the phase of speech sound acquisition where the child retracks in the hopes of reducing error factors may be viewed as the approximating phase. Here again unless the child possesses accurate comparator and active approximator mechanisms, sound learning may be affected.

Speech Sound, Zero Error. The presence of a zero error signal, as described in Chapter Two, indicates that the operations of a speech system are error-free. With respect to speech sound acquisition, the accomplishment of speech sound, zero error would mean that the child had oriented toward a particular speech sound, scanned it, tracked it, compared the model sound with his version of it, identified error factors, engaged approximating mechanisms, and, finally, successfully reproduced the model sound. From this point on, and at least for some time during childhood, the error-free speech sound is maintained via audioregulatory mechanisms. However, in time, it is believed that tactile and proprioceptive sensations begin to contribute to an increasing degree to speech sound control.

IRREGULAR SPEECH SOUND ACQUISITION

For more standard descriptions and reviews of pertinent literature on articulatory problems, the reader is referred to chapters by Van Riper and Irwin (1958, Ch. 1-4), West (1957, Ch. 6), and Berry and Eisenson (1956, Ch. 5-8).

Irregular Orienting and Looping. As already mentioned, factors which might interfere with the auditory orienting sequence toward the source of speech sounds might very well cause problems in the accurate acquisition of these sounds. Therefore, attention might be given to whether or not the auditory startle, staring, searching, and localizing sequence has taken place. The experiencing of this sequence by the child might have been affected because of a deficiency in environmental sound stimulation, or because of unpleasantness associated with the source of sound, or because of some incapacity in the child's auditory mechanism.

A significant factor, with respect to future standard sound production, is the closing of internal and external audiovocal loops during approximately the first year of life. More descriptively, the developing speaker should first show some auditory reaction to his own vocalizations, possibly by facial expressions or transient eye immobilization; he should then manifest further internal, audiovocal loop closing by his repetition of self-produced sounds; and, finally, he should manifest the completed closing of both internal and external audiovocal loops by his accurate imitation of environmental speech sounds. In the future more attention should be paid to whether the closing of such audiovocal loop processes has occurred so that certain articulatory problems may be better understood.

Irregular Scanning. At least two types of problems may occur in the scanning process. First, the scanning of environmental speech sounds might be defective for various reasons and the child may be less capable of exploring and selectively bringing to his own attention those acoustical-temporal characteristics which distinguish one speech sound from another. Second, the scanning of self-produced speech sounds may be inefficient for various reasons and the child may be less capable of exploring and selectively bringing to his own attention those acoustical-temporal characteristics which clearly distinguish one speech sound from another as produced by himself.

The more common problems of lack of experience, motivation, and problems in auditory acuity, discrimination, and span may all be recognized as possible contributors to scanning deficits. However, it is believed that more attention should be paid to the functions of auditory exploration and selection. For example, if adequate hearing, experience, and so on, exists, but, if for one reason or another, activities connected with specific auditory exploration and selection have "low energy," accurate speech sound scanning may not take place. Reasons for the possibility of such "auditory disinterest" are unclear at this time but should be investigated for and taken into account during therapy activities.

Irregular Tracking. Attempts by the child at reproducing speech events may also show deficits. If all usual factors are again equal, namely, hearing, the peripheral speech mechanism, and so on, why is it that some children do not show an inclination to engage in, or to engage in well, echoic, slave, or imagery tracking?

As in the case of scanning behavior, there may be, for reasons yet unclear, less motivation in certain children when it comes to imitative or repetitive behavior. So that in terms of the imitation of coordinated movements in general, the child's eupraxic tendencies may reflect low energy; or, in terms of speech sounds in particular, his "eulalic" or echolalic tendencies may reflect low energy. Therefore, if speech imitative tendencies are weak, little auditory tracking may be initiated; or, if repetitive tendencies are weak, there may be an inadequate amount of re-tracking in order to accurately reproduce a given speech sound. Further, and ideally for speech sound learning purposes, tracking activity should be engaged by the child not only after a given speech act (echoic) but also during the act (i.e., the child either with soft voice or silently should attempt to match the movements of the speaker's articulators with his own). Also important is the inclination toward auditory imagery tracking; in certain children, only tendencies toward echoic tracking may be present, and, consequently, there may be some difficulty in accurate speech sound learning. With respect to diagnosis and therapy for articulation problems, then, it would be important for the clinician to investigate for tracking problems, and, if such problems are found, to be prepared to devise methods for stimulating various types of tracking behavior.

Irregular Comparing. The speech sound comparing process consists of a child's comparing of a particular heard speech-sound with his self-produced version of it. Such comparing behavior may take place after the speech sound has been heard, or almost simultaneously with its production.

Speech sound comparing functions may be inefficient for at least two reasons: The first reason is connected with the inability of a particular child to determine the existence of error-factors after comparing his self-produced sound with the model sound—for example, due to reduced auditory discrimination capacity. The second reason has to do with the integrity of a function which is generally referred to as auditory memory span. It is believed that for accurate and efficient speech sound comparing to take place, the child must possess a speech perception-integration system which is capable of well-defined and adequate auditory persistence or after-hearing ability. With respect to visual stimuli, this phenomenon has been designated as after-image and refers to a visual impresson which lasts after the actual image is no longer visible. Such after-sensation phenomena may be experienced for other stimuli as well, for example, after-movement, after-taste, after-touch, and after-smell phenomena. In all these cases, what is being described is the phenomena of continuance of sensation within an individual after the eliciting stimulus has ceased.

With respect to speech sound comparing, then, it is conjectured that individuals possess differing capacities in the forming of after-impressions and that this affects their comparing functioning and, consequently, their tracking performances. Again, in terms of diagnostic procedures, it might be well for the clinician to devise means for testing for after-impression capacity (not only along auditory dimensions). As for therapy procedures, the clinician might consider developing techniques for stimulating after-sound, or after-touch, or after-movement sensitivity.

Irregular Approximating. Approximating refers to that process whereby the child, after comparing a heard sound with his own version of it, identifies error factors and, as a result, utilizes corrective tracking procedures in order to reduce these error factors.

Again, there will be found children who will not persevere in approximating procedures even when error factors have been identified; in other words, children may be found who disengage their approximator mechanisms prematurely. Reasons for such premature cessation of approximating activities by any particular child is not clear. However, this tendency should be carefully investigated for during the diagnostic session and, where appropriate, therapy activities might be designed to counteract this tendency.

Irregular, Speech-sound Zero Error. Just as the previously-described speech system irregularities are interrelated and interdependent, so too, is the concept of irregular, speech-sound zero error related and dependent on orienting, scanning, tracking, comparing, and approximating functions. For example, if there is inefficient scanning, there may be generated false zero error signals, and, therefore, this leads to a cessation of further approximating procedures which, in turn, leads to the retention of an error sound. However, the main point to be made here has to do with a speech system which performs normally and which presents appropriate error signals to the speech product corrector devise, but where there is rapid accommodation rather than progressive reduction of these error signals; and, therefore, where there are, in time, false zero error signals associated with a particular sound product. Why this rapid adaptation to error signals may take place within any particular individual deserves study and should certainly be considered during diagnostic and therapy procedures.

Many of the therapy suggestions presented above will be elaborated upon in the next section of the chapter which is devoted to therapy procedures.

There have been at least two previous and independent attempts at describing articulation therapy from the standpoint of feedback theory. Van Riper and Irwin (1958, Ch. 6) discussed the concept of scanning, and the processes of comparing and correcting in articulation therapy. The present author (Mysak, 1959) also outlined articulation therapy by utilizing a servo theory orientation. The major purpose of the present author's article was to discuss the speech system in terms of servosystem theory, basing the discussion on an extension of Fairbanks' (1954) speaking system, so that certain therapy concepts could be presented A comparison of the discussion of therapy concepts in the aforementioned article with the discussion below will reveal certain differences; these differences have come about as a result of the author's further testing of and clinical experience with these ideas.

THERAPY STAGE ONE: ACTIVATE ERROR-SOUND SENSITIVITY AND ERROR-SOUND MEASURING PROCESSES

As has been stated, closed-loop systems are error sensitive, error measuring, self-adjusting, goal-directed mechanisms. Therefore, the first stage in the adjustment of the articulatory system is to activate error-sensitivity and error-measuring processes. Following are some suggestions on how this might be done.

Error-sound Sensitivity. One of the first steps in the "orthophonemic" process is to introduce into the speech system what may be termed a therapeutic error signal (TES). The word "therapeutic" precedes the phrase since the clinician is expected to do more than simply state, "You're not making your [s] sound correctly." The client undoubtedly has heard that phrase or similar ones before. There are at least two ways in which a clinician may introduce a TES: Depending on the age of the client, the clinician should first discuss the reason why the client is coming for therapy. The obvious purpose of such a discussion is to make sure the client is aware of the purpose of his attendance (which is not always the case), and to indicate to the client that a speech specialist has now acknowledged both the presence of an error sound and the need for professional service. Specific identification of the error phoneme or phonemes should also take place during the discussion. Even though such information was undoubtedly conveyed to the client following the evaluation session, a review of such information is desirable in the initial phase of therapy. In addition to this straightforward discussion of the presence of an error sound, the clinician might reinforce the initiation of a TES by periodically demonstrating the client's error sound during the course of the initial conversations. Such demonstration activity is also instructive to the clinician since it may help the clinician determine the degree of error-sound awareness possessed by the client—at least as shown when the error sound is produced by others.

After informing the client of his error sound by discussion and demonstration, the clinician must then determine how motivated the client is for replacing his error sound with a standard sound. Again, depending on the age of the client, the clinician may plan to stimulate either extrinsic or intrinsic forms of motivation for sound modification. Extrinsic motivation may revolve about the realization by the client that error-sound correction may mean that his grades in school may improve; his job opportunities may increase, his social life may be affected, and so on. Whereas, intrinsic motivation for error-sound correction is that based on the desire to possess accurate speech for the sake of accurate speech and for the sake of communication efficiency. In the article previously mentioned (Mysak, 1959), this phase of therapy was described as the priming phase, or the preparing of the client to modify his error-sound production in the direction of the clinician's version of the sound.

These rather obvious first steps by the clinician of making sure that the client knows that there is professional confirmation of his error-sound production; of making clear which is the error sound; and of making every effort to activate all the client's motivation toward error-sound modification should not be slighted. Frequently, unsatisfactory client response to later therapy techniques is based on the clinician's having given inadequate attention to the above factors.

Error-sound Measuring. The specific goal under error-sound measuring is to intensify the therapeutic error signal so that error-sound production begins to disrupt or short circuit the automaticity of error-sound production. In terms of the components and functions of the cybernetic analogue of the speech system (Figure 1) presented in Chapter Two, the clinician must disturb the speech product comparator's predicted zero error signal, which is sent to the phase 2 transmitter, and which allows speech sound command signals issued by the phase 2 transmitter to flow rapidly without feedback monitoring because of the anticipation of error-free sound products. In other words, the clinician must devise techniques which will cause the product comparator to no longer associate a zero error with certain phonemic production; and which will cause the phase 2 transmitter to no longer automatically process or transmit certain phonemic production; and which will alert the product corrector devise for future operation. This break in the automaticity of error-sound production by the transmitter unit is of utmost importance to the success of the orthophonemic process.

The present author has already indicated (Mysak, 1959) that one way to activate error-sound measuring is by utilizing the concept of matrix analysis or standard comparisons. Such error sound-correct sound analyzing or comparing is designed to point up the differences or error factors between the client's and the clinician's phoneme production. Since sounds have auditory, visual, tactile, and kinesthetic dimensions, comparisons among all these dimensions may be made. Even though most authorities agree that the auditory channel is the most important for speech sound learning and control, the other channels quickly become important, especially in terms of speech sound control; and, therefore, it should prove worthwhile if all these dimensions are given some attention during the analysis procedure. In short, the clinician presents the standards for the different dimensions mentioned, separately or in various combinations, and compares them with the client's error-sound dimensions in the hopes of accentuating the type and degree of error being made by the client. Below are examples of procedures for correct sound-error sound analysis, or error-sound measuring of three speech sound dimensions.

Auditory Dimension. In terms of the auditory channel, Van Riper and Irwin (1958, Ch. 6) have outlined procedures for auditory scanning and comparing of correct and incorrect sounds which fit well here. Briefly, the techniques are designed to enable the child to first identify correct and incorrect versions of his sound (e.g., in syllabic, word, phrase or sentence form) as produced by the clinician (interpersonal scanning), and then to identify the error sound as it is produced by himself (intrapersonal scanning). During the auditory comparing phase of therapy, techniques are utilized ". . . by which the case comes to compare and contrast his own defective sound with the correct sound demanded by society." (Van Riper and Irwin, 1958, p. 131). It is recommended that the reader review this pertinent material.

Visual Dimension. Analysis of the visual dimension of error and standard sounds should also be done in order to amplify the TES and to ensure more accurate error measuring (especially when the error phoneme has a rather easily discernible visible component). On the environmental feedforward or clinician's side, first the visual dimension of the standard sound may be demonstrated and compared with the visual dimension of the error sound (e.g., in the case of a lateral lisp the more normal mouth posture can be compared with the common jaw lateralization and lip depression associated with lateral sound emission). Activities could then be planned where, for example, the client is asked to signal when he observes the occurrence of the error visual dimension during the time the clinician is mouthing (without voice) a list of words containing the sound under study. Of course, as this activity is pursued, the client also becomes thoroughly familiar with the error-free visual dimension of the sound under study. Such identification of visual error signals by the client should then be required during longer speech units including conversational patterns.

Such environmental error measuring of the sound pattern is important only if it contributes to the more important next step—namely, internal loop, feedback error measuring of the visual dimension. Unless the visual error factor becomes a part of the internal feedback loop (in the form of visual imagery) it serves no real purpose. One way of attempting to infuse the visual error factor into the internal feedback loop is by having the client mirror-speak without voice. Again, prepared material could be mouthed by the client, for example, memorized lines or silent repetition after the clinician, and each time the client observes the visual error factor, he is asked to signal. Another technique would involve the client's exaggeration of the articulatory posture of the error sound, thus exaggerating the visual error factor. Silent filming (videotape—if such apparatus is available) of the client during error-sound production could also be used to good advantage in helping the client evaluate the visual error factor.

Still another technique involves the client's echoing of prepared material uttered by the clinician while continuing to scrutinize the clinician's articulators. As the client begins to utter the error sound, the clinician, without voice, provides the client with simultaneous feedback of either the correct visual dimension, or the error visual dimension. The client is asked to indicate which. Here, we have a technique which provides for simultaneous comparing of the visual dimension.

Tactile-proprioceptive Dimension. The isolating of tactile-proprioceptive error factors is essential since speech sound monitoring via touch and movement sensations is believed to become more important following the speech sound learning period.

With respect to interpersonal activities, the clinician could place the client's fingers in the appropriate area of his (the clinician's) articulators while he produces the necessary movements for correct and incorrect sound production. This can be done without voice and with the client looking away from the articulators. The task of the client would be to eventually detect tactile (through the fingertips) error factors. After successfully detecting error clues as provided by the clinician, the client, by feeling his articulators with his own fingertips, could then learn to detect the tactile error factors as produced by himself.

Following these procedures, simultaneous comparing of tactile error factors can be experienced by the client, by having the client place one hand on the articulators of the clinician and one hand on his own articulators. The clinician and client may then read, simultaneously, lists of words containing error sounds without voice, and the clinician may periodically provide error or correct tactile clues for the client to detect.

Another technique for measuring the tactile-proprioceptive error factor involves silent slave speaking on the part of the client. In other words, the client slave speaks a list of error words simultaneously with the clinician. The clinician varies his correct and incorrect production of the sound and the client attempts to duplicate exactly the articulatory contacts and movements. By so doing, it is hoped the client will be able to further differentiate the tactile-proprioceptive error factors.

Such techniques should increase error-sound sensitivity within the client and should help him to become aware of, and to measure better all the dimensions of the error sound.

Error-sound Short Circuiting. The important goal of the error-sound sensitivity and error-sound measuring steps is disruption in the automatic processing by the phase 2 transmitter of words containing error sounds. Expressed in another way, the above techniques are aimed at causing the speech product comparator to predict error rather than error-free production, with reference to the sound being corrected, and thus disturb automaticity of error-sound production.

Error-sound short circuiting is an essential result of stage one therapy, and hence the clinician must be sure that the short circuiting has taken place before moving on to stage two. Signs of such short circuiting may be exhibited by the client in the form of negative facial expressions in response to his error-sound productions; or, the client may actually state that he is aware of and annoyed by his error sound as he speaks.

THERAPY STAGE TWO: ACTIVATE CORRECT-SOUND SEEKING AND APPROXIMATING AND CORRECT-SOUND TRACKING

In some cases, if all goes well, stage one procedures may activate the speech product corrector device and articulatory homeostasis may occur. However, because of various reasons, for example, severity of the problem and age of the client, this does not happen frequently enough and further speech sound guidance may have to be given.

Correct-sound Seeking and Approximating. Correct-sound seeking and approximating behavior should follow rather spontaneously error-sound short-circuiting. That is, once error-sound sensitivity, error-measuring, and error-sound short-circuiting processes have been activated, the client's product corrector device should begin making attempts at speech sound readjustment. In other words, the speech system should make efforts at eliminating the newly-infused error signals associated with the production of a specific error sound.

Speech-sound seeking and approximating may be encouraged by simply requesting the client to experiment with the production of his error sound. He might be asked, for example, to attempt to make the sound in as many different ways as possible during the course of a conversation; this request

is made in order to facilitate his attempts at progressively reducing associated error factors. To encourage such seeking and approximating activities,
the client may be asked to imitate how a little boy, or a grown girl, or his
teacher, and so on, makes that particular sound. The point behind such
activities is to encourage the client to produce the sound undergoing modification with as many different auditory, visual, and tactile-proprioceptive
dimensions as possible, so that one combination may be found which will
generate the smallest number of error signals. During these attempts the
clinician should, of course, reinforce those versions of the sound which
come close to the standard product. Seeking and approximating behavior
should go on until the client's error sound is produced more and more in-
consistently. This type of activity is engaged in before more direct attempts
are made at getting the client to produce the correct sound.

Correct-sound Tracking. Again, it is hoped that seeking-approximating
work will eventually result in correct sound production. If this is not the
case, tracking techniques are tried next. It should be emphasized that the
goal of therapy up to this point is to have achieved correction before therapeutic tracking techniques become necessary.

Corrective tracking includes the following four steps: (1) The client
is informed that he will be asked to attempt directly the reproduction of
the correct sound. (2) The clinician decides on the most appropriate combination of correct sound dimensions to present to his particular client. In
this regard, the clinician may have found that during the error-measuring
procedures, the client was most responsive to one particular sound dimension or some particular combination of sound dimensions. So that in some
cases, the clinician may choose to present the auditory-visual dimensions
of the sound (the ones usually exposed to the child during the speech learning period); or, he may choose to present the auditory, visual, and tactile-
proprioceptive dimensions (a synesthetic approach); or, he may choose,
again because of his particular client, to eliminate certain dimensions, for
example, he may choose to present only the auditory dimension, or only
the visual, or only visual plus tactile-proprioceptive dimensions (individual
stimulus complex approach). (3) The clinician then requests the client to
carefully scan for the particular sound dimension or dimensions about to
be exhibited so that when asked he (the client) may be able to track the
sound accurately. (4) After stimulating the client until the client indicates
he feels able to track well, the clinician allows the client to make his attempt. During the client's first attempt at correct sound production, the
clinician should make every effort to guide the client toward correct sound
production by continuing to provide auditory and visual clues and by actually guiding the articulators, if necessary. As stated previously (Mysak,
1959), such procedures allow minimal error signals to be fed back into the
system, thus accentuating the previously determined error factors and also

increasing the chances for further refinement of correct sound production.

Correct-sound Automaticity. After the correct sound has been accurately tracked by the client, the clinician must usually plan for ways of helping the client to integrate the new sound into his conversational patterns. Of course, it is hoped that once successful tracking has taken place, the client may experience rather spontaneous error sensitive, error measuring, self-adjusting articulatory behavior; but, again, this unfortunately is not the usual case. Correct-sound automaticity techniques must proceed until the time the speech product comparator is predicting error-free production of the corrected sound, and the product corrector devise is only needed to handle transient errors.

Repetition of production of the correct sound (practicing the sound in isolation, in syllabic form, and in semantic form such as in words, phrases, sentences, stories, and in conversations in and out of the therapy room) is one way of moving toward the goal of automaticity of production of the correct sound. Other techniques include negative practice work where the client is asked to intentionally produce error signals in order to ensure proper operation of the speech product comparator and corrector; and imagery speech feedback work where the client is asked to practice the correct sound with his mind's articulators. It is expected that imagery work would also exert positive influences on the speech product comparator and corrector devices.

SUMMARY

1. Normal speech sound acquisition is described and involves the following sequence: auditory orienting to, and scanning, tracking, comparing, and approximating of, environmental speech sounds.

2. Some reasons for abnormal speech sound development are presented. Problems in orienting and looping, and of irregular scanning, tracking, comparing, and approximating activities are discussed.

3. Two stages in articulation therapy are outlined. The first stage of therapy involves the activation of error-sound sensitivity and error-measuring processes and the short-circuiting of the automatic production of the error sound; the second stage of therapy involves the activation of correct-sound seeking and approximating and correct-sound tracking processes and the establishment of automaticity of correct sound production.

REFERENCES

BERRY, MILDRED, F., and EISENSON, J.: *Speech Disorders: Principles and Practices of Therapy.* New York, Appleton, 1956.

FAIRBANKS, G.: Systematic research in experimental phonetics: 1. A theory of the speech mechanism as a servosystem. *J. Speech Hearing Dis., 19*:133-139, 1954.

McCurry, W. H., and Irwin, O. C.: A study of word approximations in the spontaneous speech of infants. *J. Speech Hearing Dis.*, *18*:133-139, 1953.

Mysak, E. D.: A servo model for speech therapy. *J. Speech Hearing Dis.*, *24*:144-149, 1959.

Van Riper, C., and Irwin, J. V.: *Voice and Articulation*. Englewood Cliffs, Prentice-Hall, 1958.

West, R., Ansberry, M., and Carr, Anna: *The Rehabilitation of Speech*. New York, Harper, 1957.

Chapter Seven

TONAL FLOW

SPEECH FLUENCY, or tonal flow, is the subject of the final chapter of the book. The plan of the chapter is to discuss the developmental sequence of the regulation of tonal flow, the symptoms and possible causes of abnormal tonal flow, and some therapy procedures for these symptoms.

DEVELOPMENTAL SEQUENCE OF TONAL FLOW REGULATION

As an introduction to the discussion of the development of tonal flow regulation, it would be useful to review the findings of Metraux (1950). Metraux studied the pronunciation, voice, repetition, and language of children at ages 18, 24, 30, 36, 42, 48, and 54 months. For purposes of this section, only her findings with respect to developmental repetition will be described.

Following are Metraux's findings on changes in fluency in the child from 18 to 54 months. At 18 months: The child may be observed to repeat "syllables or words more frequently than not." The "repetition is easy, unforced repetition which can be terminated by himself or by the response of others." At 24 months: The child now uses "[ʌ] before many responses . . ." and ". . . may repeat [ʌʌ] before he finds the correct response." The child may repeat "I" before answering questions and there is occasional syllable repetition. ". . . The most common characteristic of repetition at this age is a kind of compulsive repetition of a word or phrase." In some children, there were as many as six or seven such repetitions, in others, there were only two. At 30 months: "The compulsive repetition of a phrase is even more marked now than at 24 months." Some children were observed to ". . . continue interminably with more force, higher pitch and volume each time." Further, Metraux indicated that at 24 months the repetition seemed to be caused by internal factors, while at 30 months, because of the child's greater use of speech for intercommunication purposes, external factors may often be observed to cause an increase in repetition. In addition, the child at this time "demands repetition from others" for example, with respect to wanting stories and poems repeated. ". . . Developmental stuttering is usually evidenced for the first time at this age." According to Metraux, this developmental stuttering is characterized by repetition of the first word or syllable with the repetition often progressing to a tonic block; however, this block is easily broken and gives the child no great dif-

[84]

ficulty. At 36 months: "Most children are again on an easy repetitive basis with none of the compulsion noted earlier." When answering questions, he may occasionally echo phrases between performances. Further, ". . . occasional repetition of the beginning syllable, an [ʌ] or [ʌm] is often used as a starter for speech." Some instances of medial sound repetitions are observed, but tonic blocks on initial syllables are infrequent. At 42 months: "Repetitions are frequent and occur with almost every child." It again has "a somewhat compulsive quality as it did at 30 months." Unlike the 30 month stage, however, these repetitions may often be terminated by introducing a new subject or object. Further, the repetition is frequently ". . . related to another person, in demand for attention, information or encouragement." ". . . Developmental stuttering is again prominent and is often characterized by a tonic block on the initial syllable, the duration of which is usually longer than at 30 months." Speech blocking at this time may also be accompanied by grimacing, cocking the head, and so forth. Rate of speech also appears faster at this time. At 48 months: "There is little repetition at this age in comparison to some of the preceding ages." Phrasal repetitions are heard occasionally but without the "compulsive quality." However, the child who has previously shown signs of developmental stuttering may continue to have repetition and blocking episodes. Finally, at 54 months: The child often uses [ʌm] or [ʌ] "in a musing fashion at the beginning of a phrase, but he repeats seldom except for emphasis." The child who has earlier shown speech blocking may again show occasional difficulty. ". . . If he blocks now, it is probably characterized by a slower rate, with a long breath before he starts to speak."

Certain findings by Davis (1939, 1940) are also pertinent to this discussion. Investigation of 62 nonstuttering children aged two to five revealed that: repetition is common to all children, but the amount and kind of repetition differs among children; repetition of words and phrases decreased with age but syllable repetitions appeared unaffected by age; at all ages, syllable repetitions occurred less frequently than either word or phrase repetitions; instances of syllable repetition and the number of such repetitive syllables ". . . were the best measures for determining the children who deviated markedly from the group. In each of these measures the child who was termed a 'stutterer' stands out dramatically from the balance of the group."

Finally, Wingate's (1962) review of the literature of speech characteristics of young children further contributes to the purpose of this section of the chapter. In a summary statement, Wingate indicates: "First it seems evident that children do show considerable individual variation in the type, amount, and frequency of their fluency irregularities. Second, certain kinds of fluency irregularities are found much more frequently in children 'identified as stutterers' and also are quite consistently identified as not normal . . ." The irregularities referred to are considered to be predominantly those of syllable repetitions and prolongations.

The findings reported above contribute to the following concepts regarding the developmental sequence of tonal flow regulation: (1) There is a development from internal loop, feedforward-feedback instability and control over tonal flow to external loop, feedforward-feedback control over tonal flow. In other words, there is first control over internal factors which contribute to tonal flow irregularity such as immature association circuits between percept, heard word, and spoken word-patterns; and then control over external factors which contribute to tonal flow irregularity such as attempts at gaining a listener's attention, or the fear of losing his attention, or interruptions by the listener. This sequence from internal loop to external loop control is in keeping with other developmental sequences presented in Chapter Three. (2) Automaticity of utterances of articulatory cycles proceeds from syllabic, to word, to phrasal, to full cycle levels. (3) Interference with the progressive regulation of speech automaticity may be reflected by an arrestation at the phonemic or syllabic level of automaticity.

SYMPTOMS OF IRREGULAR TONAL FLOW

When for one reason or another tonal flow regulation does not proceed normally, certain rather common symptoms become discernible. With regard to developing symptomatology, Bloodstein (1960a, 1960b, 1961) recently described four phases of stuttering. In brief, they are: (1) the preschool stage marked by episodic repetitions at the beginning of sentences and on minor parts of speech with little evidence of concern shown by the child; (2) the early elementary school stage marked by chronic blocks on major parts of speech with the child still showing little or no concern about his blocks, but with the child now regarding himself as a stutterer; (3) the junior high and high school stage marked by stuttering occurrence chiefly in response to specific situations, and the appearance of sound and word precipitators and the use of word substitutions and circumlocutions with essentially no avoidance of speaking situations and little or no evidence of fear or embarrassment; and, finally, (4) the high school and older stage marked by strong anticipation of stuttering, feared sounds, words, and situations, and frequent use of word substitutions and circumlocutions with avoidance of speech situations and other evidences of fear and embarrassment. Bloodstein emphasizes that the phases are variable, typical rather than universal, and that the changes are continuous and gradual. Again, for purposes of our discussion, it is interesting to note that in Bloodstein's developmental phases, the major source of difficulty for the individual appears to be on an internal basis during the beginning phases of his problem, and becomes increasingly more affected by external or environmental factors during the later phases.

It may be conjectured, then, that each child possesses an individual capacity for tonal flow regulation and that each child's speech automaticity mechanism matures at a particular rate. It may be conjectured further that if a particular child responds to his speech automaticity level in a negative fashion, or if significant others do, the child, whose speech automaticity maturation may either be proceeding normally, or whose automaticity maturation may be showing signs of interference, may develop the complex of symptoms commonly identified as stuttering. The point being made here is that, whether or not there are actual differences in automaticity mechanisms, the kinds of symptoms usually associated with stuttering may, for the most part, be based on childish reactions to either a within or a without normal limits speech automaticity mechanism.

Irregular Motor Reaction. In their simplest form, tonal flow irregularities may be seen as increases in the amount of sound or syllable repetitions or prolongations, or as increases in the number of such repetitions or prolongations per speech cycle. There is also the possibility, of course, that the development of the child's tonal flow capacity may be within the normal range, but that these normal flow irregularities may be misinterpreted as being abnormal, in accordance with the theory of Johnson (1957). In either case, the child may eventually become concerned with his level of speech automaticity and may attempt to reduce the number or frequency of syllable repetitions or prolongations. The child's efforts at increasing his level of speech automaticity at a time when he may be neurophysiologically unable to, usually succeeds in only further reducing it. The child's motor reactions to actual or inferred tonal flow irregularities may be divided into the following two categories.

Articulatory Movements and Feedback. In response to developmental irregularities in tonal flow, the child may attempt either to reduce the number of syllable repetitions or to reduce the syllable prolongation time—again, at a time when such goals may not be within his neurophysiological capacity. Repeated attempts at assuming a more mature basal fluency level frequently results in increasing muscle tone during syllable repetitions, thereby giving some syllables a clonic characteristic; and in increasing muscle tone during syllable prolongations, thereby giving other syllables a tonic characteristic. Further, a reverberating circuit may develop from the child's over-innervation of his articulators and the consequent increase in tactile, pressure, and proprioceptive feedbacks from these articulators. That is, as the child attempts to reduce the number of repetitions or the prolongation time of certain phonemes or syllables by using excessive muscle action, the amplified sensory feedbacks from his peripheral speech mechanism may develop further speech anxiety within the child which, in turn, may generate even stronger outflows of motor impulses to the articulatory mechanism. To further complicate the situation, as this articulatory sensorimotor reverberating circuit develops, there may be nervous irradiation from the articulators to the surrounding muscles of the face, head, and neck, and the commonly observed facial grimacing, eye blinking, forehead creasing, alar flaring, head bending, and so on, may appear. The accompanying sensory feedback from these overflow movements may then, in turn, also contribute to the strength of the articulatory sensorimotor reverberating circuit.

Circuit-breaking Motor Activities and Feedback. To further complicate this self-generated motor abnormality, the affected individual may begin to acquire what might be called circuit-breaking motor patterns. For example, he may find that if he quickly swings his body in a forward direction at the initiation of the reverberating circuit, he breaks the circuit and the flow of speech continues until the next moment of difficulty. Again, the clinician may recognize many forms of these circuit breakers such as the foot stamp, arm swing, finger press, and leg swing. Unfortunately, for the affected individual, circuit-breaking activities: (1) usually add to the unusual speech-associated motor activities; (2) may be tolerated eventually by the speech system and thereby lose their effectiveness; and (3) may eventually contribute sensory feedback energy of their own into the reverberating circuit.

Irregular Perceptual-conceptual Reactions. In addition to the irregular motor reactions which contribute to as well as tend to maintain the tonal flow irregularities, there are various perceptual-conceptual reactions which tend to do the same. It should be mentioned that misperceptions and misconceptions with respect to tonal flow irregularity may arise from the individual himself; may be introjected from the environment; or more frequently, may develop as a combination of both factors.

Misperceptions about Intrinsic Speech-sound Difficulty and Feedback. Affected individuals may in time begin to perceive certain speech sounds as being more detrimental to tonal flow regularity than others. Such perceptual sets may develop because the individual recalls repeating or prolonging certain phonemes more often and with greater frequency; for example, an individual may have used a particular phoneme more frequently in situations of communicative stress. Or the phoneme, at a particular time in the child's speech sound maturation period, may actually have been more difficult for him to utter; or his attention may have been drawn to the sound when certain individuals in his environment attempted to help him utter the sound in a "smoother" fashion, and so on. Whatever the case, the important factor is that the individual perceives, or rather misperceives, the sound as possessing some kind of inherent flow-disturbance characteristic.

As in the case of irregular motor activity, the perceptual-conceptual problem usually irradiates outwards and eventually involves types of listeners and particular situations. That is, speech flow irregularity may appear even more evident in certain situations such as during the use of the telephone, or during recitations, or when the individual speaks to authority figures.

The feedback factor is also present in the misperception-misconception aspect of the tonal flow problem. It may be readily appreciated that if an individual considers that certain sounds possess intrinsic flow-interruption characteristics, he may attempt "to get set" for those sounds and hence tend to increase the muscle tone in his articulators which, in turn, contributes to tonal flow interruption. Then, when the sounds do in actuality disturb tonal flow, there is additional feedback which strengthens the misconceptions with respect to the flow-disturbance characteristics of the sounds; it should be apparent that such perceptual-conceptual activity will also contribute further to the irregular motor reactions, and so on. In other words, a self-generating and more complicated perceptual-motor-sensory reverberating circuit usually develops and this contributes to and maintains the tonal flow problem.

Circuit-breaking Conceptual Activities and Feedback. Again to further complicate matters, the individual who develops misconceptions and becomes anxious about certain speech sounds or speaking situations may attempt to break the reverberating circuit by avoiding speaking situations entirely; by avoiding certain sounds (use of circumlocutions and synonyms); or by using commonly encountered "starters," "stallers," and so on. Again, such activity feeds back and tends to reinforce not only the misperceptions and misconceptions but the whole reverberating, tonal-flow circuitry.

Finally, the perceptual-motor-sensory reverberating circuit which disturbs tonal flow is further energized by feedback from concomitant physiological and psychological reactions. The physiological reactions accompanying speech flow interruption may include vasomotor and sudomotor reactions, changes in heart beat, respiration, and biochemistry; while the psychological reactions may include states such as anxiety, confusion, embarrassment, humiliation, guilt and shame.

The next section will be devoted to a discussion of the many places in the total speech system where involvements may manifest themselves in the form of stuttering speech behavior.

FORMS OF IRREGULAR TONAL FLOW

In a recent article (Mysak, 1960), the present writer included in his discussion the concept of verbalizing automaticity and also described loci in the speech circuitry where problems may interfere with tonal flow. These concepts are pertinent to the material presented in this section of the chapter and hence will be referred to frequently.

Verbalizing Process. Before discussing circuitry involvements which may lead to breaks in speech automaticity, it would be valuable to review briefly the automaticity mechanisms associated with the various perceptual-linguistic or verbalizing processes.

It might be recalled that in Chapter Two the speech system was described as a closed, multiple-loop system containing feedforward and feedback internal and external loops. In the internal loop aspect, automatic and reciprocal connections may be found between thought patterns and word-formation patterns; between the comparison of thought and word patterns (inner speech monitoring); between word-formation patterns and word-production patterns; and between the comparison of word production and thought patterns (outer speech monitoring). In the external loop aspect, an automatic and reciprocal connection may be found between word production and listener reaction. When all the automatic and reciprocal connections are working well, the speech system should enjoy good tonal flow or verbalizing automaticity; however, if automaticity mechanisms are disturbed in one or more of the described circuits, the speech system might reflect tonal flow irregularities or disturbances in verbalizing automaticity. It is believed that when an individual has an understanding of all the perceptual-linguistic operations that may be involved in verbalizing, and has an appreciation of the necessary automaticity mechanisms involved in these operations, the use of the term verbalizing deautomaticity becomes a more accurate way of describing tonal flow irregularities than does the use of the less meaningful term stuttering.

Loci of Disturbances in Verbalizing Automaticity. It is proposed that there may be many disturbances in automaticity mechanisms, associated with internal as well as external loop speech circuitry, which may directly or indirectly be manifested in the form of commonly recognized stuttering symptomatology. Following are examples of such automaticity disturbances.

Thought Pattern-Word Formation. Factors which may interfere with the speaker's automatic and reciprocal connections between thoughts and words include actual or mental experiences with listeners, or with listeners and situations, which may, for example, automatically elicit socially unacceptable language within the speaker. To speak or not to speak becomes a problem for the speaker because of the expected negative reactions from the environment to such undesirable language; and the speaker, therefore, feels the need to guard against the automatic processing of his thoughts into words. As an example of this type of verbalizing deautomaticity, Travis (1957, p. 919) has written, "When any person stutters, he is blocking something else besides what you and he might think he is trying to say; something else that is pressing for verbal expression but which will be intolerable to you and to him alike should it be uttered." Along these lines,

Sheehan (1958) has remarked that unexpressed hostility and verbal aggression might also be considered as factors in stuttering behavior.

Word Formation-Word Production. The automaticity mechanism in the word formation-word production circuit may be disturbed by the periodic uncontrolled release of electrical potential in areas of the brain that subserve word formulation, and in areas of the brain responsible for innervating articulatory musculature. Similar disturbances in automatic processing of speech units is manifested rather dramatically in the condition known as palilalia which is a speech disorder ". . . characterized by repetition of a phrase which the patient reiterates with increasing rapidity. It is most frequently encountered as a symptom of Parkinsonism following encephalitis lethargica and in pseudobulbar palsy due to vascular lesions (Brain, 1961, p. 106)." Penfield and Roberts (1959, p. 133), in describing some of their findings with patients receiving brain surgery for the treatment of focal epilepsy, state that hesitation, slurring, distortion and repetition of words may occur when various areas of the brain are interfered with by electrical stimulation. Finally, West (1958, Ch. 4) has recently written that the fundamental disorder of stuttering may very well be related to pyknolepsy and may be referred to as "phemolepsy" or "speech epilepsy."

Word Production-Anticipation of Fluency of Word Production. The third break in tonal flow automaticity may occur upon the development within the speech product comparator of a predicted fluency error signal. This development may take place because of at least two reasons: First, if parents, relatives, or friends emit signals rather regularly which indicate concern over the child's fluency ability during the time his speech may be characterized by developmental syllable, word, and phrasal repetitions, these negative signals may eventually arouse concern within the child about his own fluency ability and this concern, in turn, may contribute to the development of a disfluency rather than a fluency prediction in the child's speech product comparator. In other words, abnormal tonal flow may occur when significant others regularly over-monitor and are critical of the child's normal tonal flow, and when eventually the child introjects this over-monitoring tendency and becomes over-critical of his own tonal flow (after Johnson). Second, a similar series of events may occur if the child actually does suffer from an abnormal number and frequency of syllable repetitions and he himself becomes concerned over his tonal flow capacity and begins to anticipate problems with it.

Word Production-Thought Pattern Comparison. Automaticity of word production-thought pattern comparison describes that process by which speakers automatically scan the adequacy or correctness of the symbols they are transmitting to listeners. Hence, any disturbance in the return of these signals back to the speaker may disturb tonal flow. As indicated in Chapter One, numerous investigators have indicated that one effect of delaying the normal auditory feedback of speakers is to produce rate and rhythm changes in their speech which may simulate stuttering. Further, it may be recalled Stromsta found that one of the rather consistent effects of distorting air-conducted feedback to a speaker was to induce blockage of phonation. Finally, Tomatis (1963, Ch. 6), in writing about the dominant ear and the speaking voice, reported the following: When he fed back a certain speaker's voice to the speaker's left ear only, not only was the speaker's voice quality affected but the speaker also showed hesitations, "uhs," syllabic repetition and, finally, showed what Tomatis described as stuttering. In follow-up experiments, he found that this rhythm effect was quite variable and that stuttering phenomena did not consistently appear; however, he does report that there is almost always some modification in verbal flow. He reported further that he has found many stutterers who show dominant ear deficiencies and that many of these responded to therapy aimed at producing a dominant ear.

Word Production-Listener Reaction Comparison. It may be assumed that there is some type of automatic assessment on the part of a speaker of a listener's reaction to the speaker's oral message (as described in Chapter Two). In other words, for individuals to enjoy successful oral communication, they need to develop an awareness of whether or not what they are saying is actually being understood, and whether or not what they are saying is being understood in the way they intend it. For example, if a child finds that he frequently misinterprets his listener's reactions, he may begin to lose confidence in his ability to express himself and may begin to anticipate that the listener will not completely understand him. This may cause the child to habitually re-formulate or repeat his utterances and hence his speech automaticity or tonal flow may slowly be affected.

In summary, verbalizing automaticity may be affected by disturbances in automaticity mechanisms associated with the following speech circuits: thought pattern-word formation, word formation-word production, word production-anticipation of fluency of word production, word production-thought pattern comparison, and word production-listener reaction comparison. Or, stated positively and more simply, verbalizing automaticity depends on the automatic and reciprocal functioning of a series of internal and external loop speech circuits.

It should also be mentioned here that breaks in automaticity mechanisms at any point in the speech circuitry are usually compounded by repercussions at other points. For example, automaticity breaks in the thought pattern-word formation, or word formation-word production circuits will eventually lead to disturbances in the word production-anticipation of fluency of word production circuit. It is this type of chain reaction that makes it difficult for the clinician to determine the origin or origins of the automaticity involvement, and hence makes it difficult for him to plan the most efficient therapy approach to any one particular case of verbalizing deautomaticity.

The final section of the chapter will be devoted to a discussion of therapy techniques designed to re-establish speech automaticity or tonal flow regularity.

RE-AUTOMATIZATION THERAPY PROCEDURES

The techniques described below are aimed basically at relieving symptoms of tonal flow irregularity. An effort will be made to avoid repeating standard techniques for stuttering therapy such as those advanced by Van Riper (1963, Ch. 12) and Johnson (1956, Ch. 5).

Further, in the discussion of therapy techniques, the reader will find that emphasis is placed on establishing internal loop, feedforward-feedback stability and control; a goal which is in keeping with the developmental sequence of tonal flow regulation.

Diagnosis of Type of Deautomaticity. As outlined in the article previously referred to (Mysak, 1960), the first step toward planning the most effective approach to speech system re-automatization is to attempt to identify the offending circuit or circuits within the affected individual's speech circuitry. For example, if it is determined that the automaticity disturbance is connected with a thought-word formation problem, attention would have to be given to parent-child problems which may be arousing emotions such as guilt, hostility, frustration, and fear within the child and which, in turn, may be affecting his tonal flow; if the automaticity disturbance appears connected with a word formation-word production problem, the use of certain anti-convulsants may be considered during certain periods of tonal flow maturation; if the automaticity disturbance appears connected with a word production-anticipation of fluency of word production problem, pertinent information about tonal flow maturation and how this maturation may be affected can be offered to parents of children so involved; if the automaticity disturbance appears connected with a word production-thought comparison problem, attention may be given to the construction of special audicles designed to modify the speech feedback of certain individuals, or designed to establish a lead ear; finally, if the automaticity disturbance appears related to a word production-listener reaction comparison problem, work may need to be done to help the child better evaluate facial expressions and other factors which reveal how his message is being received and interpreted by his listener.

As has already been pointed out, unless the clinician observes the child experiencing his speech automaticity problems early and before the usual compounding or chaining of automaticity disturbances, it is very difficult to determine exactly the original circuit involvement. However, areas that should be investigated and which may be of some value in ascertaining the locus of the break are: family history (e.g., tissue predisposition?), age of onset, form of initial flow interruptions (e.g., syllable, word, or phrasal repetition?, associated motor problems?), conditions under which interruptions appear (e.g., when speaking to certain individuals, about certain subjects, anytime?, etc.), verbal diadochocinesis, and adaptation rate (rapid or no adaptation, presence or lack of consistency effect?).

In short, evidence should be collected which may help to identify external loop and (or) internal loop automaticity stresses, actual tonal flow irregularities or imagined irregularities, and so on.

Re-establish a Fluency, Zero Error Signal. It has been indicated that when tonal flow irregularity becomes a clinical problem, it means that a fluency error signal has developed within the speech product comparator and it is this signal which continues to affect the automaticity of the phase 2 transmitter. Hence, a major goal in a feedback-oriented therapy is to gradually weaken the strength of the fluency error signal and to re-establish within the comparator a fluency, zero error signal.

One way of helping to achieve this goal is to have the client engage in speech activities which ordinarily are free of flow agitators as often and as long as possible each day. Following are some suggestions.

Speaking Conditions. Bloodstein (1950) attempted to determine those conditions under which stutterers report their stuttering to be reduced or absent. Some of these conditions may be selected by the clinician and used to weaken the prediction of a fluency error signal within a particular client's comparator. Following are some specific examples of speaking situations in which fluency error signals are usually minimal: reading or speaking aloud in isolation, speaking to animals or infants, echo speaking, slave speaking, reading or speaking nonsense material, speaking in a sing-song manner, speaking through closed teeth, singing, choral reading, imitation of another person's manner of speaking (e.g., foreign accent, regionalism), and simultaneous speaking and writing. It should also prove useful to have the client frequently engage in mirror speaking under these positive speaking conditions so that he may associate his speaking self with speech fluency. He should also record as much of this material as possible and bathe his ears in the playback while looking at himself in the mirror.

Below are examples of additional techniques designed to facilitate fluency and hence to weaken the prediction of fluency error signals within the client's speech product comparator.

Speech Imagery Feedback. The client may be asked to practice regular tonal flow with his mind's articulators, so to speak. He may, for example, imagine himself reciting, giving a talk or holding a conversation—all in a fluent fashion.

Solo Speech Feedback. Leading one's motor activities with a running description of these motor activities (speaking to one's self) is one form of solo speech feedback. The use of monologies or soliloquies are other forms of solo speech feedback work which tend to facilitate fluency. During such work the client may be asked to describe to himself, whenever he has the opportunity, the happenings of the day up to that point, or to utter whatever comes to mind.

Attenuated Speech Feedback. In many instances, stutterers experience improvement in speech flow when their auditory feedback is reduced (Maraist and Hutton, 1957; Cherry *et al.*, 1956). Thus, if certain levels of masking noise appear to affect positively a particular client's tonal flow, he may be exposed to such therapeutic masking as often as is useful.

Steady State Fluency Error Signal. It may be remembered that steady state error signals are those which may be generated during the routine operation of the speech system (see Chapter Two). Therefore, during such routine operation the speech product comparator and corrector devices are processing in an easy fashion familiar and slight differences between desired tonal flow and actual tonal flow. On the other hand, transient error signals describe sudden variations in the operation of the speech system which usually trigger rather radical shifts in operation and hence overshooting and system oscillation activity. It is apparent that actual or assumed transient fluency error signals may lead to increased flow interruption.

Therefore, another way of contributing to the development of a fluency, zero error signal is by utilizing techniques which may reduce some of the actual or supposed transient fluency error signals to steady state fluency error signals. One approach to such speech system accommodation work is to have the client periodically produce intentional flow irregularity; this activity should eventually contribute to desensitizing his comparator and corrector devices. Another desensitization technique involves having the client frequently record and playback his own stuttered speech as well as to listen to and observe the stuttering of others.

Developmental Fluency Feedback. At the beginning of this chapter it was shown that the development of speech automaticity appears to proceed from the syllabic, to the word, to the phrasal, and, finally, to the full articulatory cycle level. Further, it was stated that individuals showing difficulty in developing speech automaticity usually reflect an arrestation at the syllabic level.

Therefore, as a technique to counteract such a developmental arrestation, it is recommended that client's be asked to frequently engage in intentional whole word and phrasal repetitions during oral reading exercises or during conversational patterns.

Shunted Speech Feedback. The concept of shunted speech feedback was discussed in Chapter Two. There it was explained that since the speech system's output is associated with more than one type of feedback, for ex-

ample, auditory, tactile, and proprioceptive feedbacks, the process of reducing the efficiency or of inactivating one or two of the feedbacks, and
thus allowing the remaining channel to become the dominant feedback
channel, may be described as shunting speech feedback.

This shunting concept has relevance to the problem of stuttering since
many stutterers appear to possess over-correcting (underdamped) auditory
monitoring systems. Such an over-sensitive monitoring channel may feed
back tonal flow error signals which are so small that they would ordinarily
be disregarded. This excessive backflow of inconsequential error-signals
over-activates the corrector device and hence speech automaticity is disturbed.

It may also be hypothesized that certain cases of tonal flow irregularity
are based on the arrestation of speech product monitoring on the auditory
level. This idea is related to the concept that during the speech sound learning period the auditory channel is the primary channel for receiving speech
signals from the environment, as well as the primary channel for monitoring self-produced oral symbols and speech sounds. It is believed that gradually, as speech systems mature, the auditory channel is used more and
more for speech symbol monitoring and that speech sound monitoring is
assumed more completely by tactile and proprioceptive channels. This
gradual separation of monitoring functions no doubt contributes to speech
proficiency. Stated in another way, it is advanced that speech output and
control are most efficient when speech content is monitored by the "thinking brain" via the ear, while speech product is monitored primarily by the
"doing brain" via the tactile and proprioceptive channels. Returning to this
paragraph's opening statement, then, some individuals may reflect flow irregularities because they have continued to monitor both speech content and product primarily with the ear and because this immature
form of speech monitoring may be inefficient for more complicated speech
output and control. If such a situation is actually contributing to flow irregularities in any particular case, shunting procedures should be helpful.

Finally, feedback shunting may be important if the primary monitoring channel or channels in any given case happen not to be functioning
well because of some type of speech system interference. Techniques for
shunting feedback follow.

Attenuated Speech Feedback. Auditory masking or auditory feedback
attenuation may be used as a shunting technique which causes the speaker
to increase his tactile and proprioceptive monitoring of his speech product.
Other techniques under this heading include either having the client completely eliminate his vocalization during articulation, that is, by having
him just move his articulators, or partially eliminating his vocalization by
having him whisper. Again, both techniques are designed to accentuate
the speech control functions of touch and movement feedbacks.

Amplified Speech Feedback. In line with the above technique, if the auditory channel is found to be a speech flow agitator and it appears desirable to shunt the monitoring function to touch-movement feedback channels, such touch-movement feedbacks may be amplified by having the client intentionally focus on these sensations during his articulatory activity. Or, he may be asked to exaggerate his articulatory movements, or to feel his articulators as they move, or to watch them as they move, or to move them against resistence created by his own fingers (e.g., pressing against the lips, holding the mandible, etc.).

Double Speech Feedback. It was stated in Chapter Two that double speech feedback may occur if an individual watches closely the articulators of a lead speaker and attempts to track simultaneously the words of the lead speaker. Hence, simultaneous tracking results in the tracker receiving environmental visual and auditory signals while simultaneously receiving his own auditory, tactile, and proprioceptive feedbacks. Such activity should contribute to the shunting goal since the speech tracker must concentrate on the visual signals from the lead speaker's articulatory movements and on his own tactile and proprioceptive feedbacks.

SUMMARY

1. The development of tonal flow regulation is described. In short, it is shown that speech flow development is marked by first control over internal loop factors which contribute to flow irregularity, and then by control over external loop factors which contribute to tonal flow irregularity.

2. Symptoms of irregular tonal flow are cited and include irregular motor and perceptual-conceptual reactions.

3. Automaticity breaks in at least five circuits of the speech system are identified as contributing to tonal flow disturbances. The circuits involved are: thought pattern-word formation, word formation-word production, word production-anticipation of fluency of word production, word production-thought pattern comparison, and word production-listener reaction comparison.

4. Procedures for re-automatizing tonal flow are outlined and include techniques designed to develop a fluency, zero error signal in the speech product comparator, and techniques for shunting speech-product feedback monitoring to tactile and proprioceptive channels.

With the close of this chapter the story of the book comes to a beginning rather than to an end. It is hoped that the ideas presented will stimulate new thinking about speech theory, speech disorders, and speech therapy and, consequently, serve as points of departure for many new researches. When all is done, an idea is good if it stimulates productive thinking and it has been said that productive thinking may well start with the consideration of possible analogies.

REFERENCES

BLOODSTEIN, O.: The development of stuttering: I. Changes in nine basic features. *J. Speech Hearing Dis.*, 25:219-237, 1960.

BLOODSTEIN, O.: The development of stuttering: II. Developmental phases. *J. Speech Hearing Dis.*, 25:366-376, 1960.

BLOODSTEIN, O.: The development of stuttering: III. Theoretical and clinical implications. *J. Speech Hearing Dis.*, 26:67-82, 1961.

BLOODSTEIN, O.: A rating scale study of conditions under which stuttering is reduced or absent. *J. Speech Hearing Dis.*, 15:29-36, 1950.

BRAIN, R.: *Speech Disorders*. Washington, Butterworth, 1961.

CHERRY, C., SAYERS, B., and MARLAND, PAULINE: Experiments upon the total inhibition of stammering by external control and some clinical results. *J. Psychosom. Res.*, 1:233-246, 1956.

DAVIS, D. M.: The relation of repetitions in the speech of young children to certain measures of language maturity and situational factors: Part I. *J. Speech Dis.*, 4:303-318, 1939.

DAVIS, D. M.: The relation of repetitions in the speech of young children to certain measures of language maturity and situational factors: Part II and Part III. *J. Speech Dis.*, 5:235-246, 1940.

JOHNSON, W., et al.: *Speech Handicapped School Children*. New York, Harper, 1956.

JOHNSON, W.: Perceptual and evaluational factors in stuttering. In: *Handbook of Speech Pathology*, L. E. Travis, Ed. New York, Appleton, 1957.

MARAIST, JEAN ANN, and HUTTON, C.: Effects of auditory masking upon the speech of stutterers. *J. Speech Hearing Dis.*, 22:385-389, 1957.

METRAUX, RUTH W.: Speech profiles of the pre-school child 18 to 54 months. *J. Speech Hearing Dis.*, 15:37-53, 1950.

MYSAK, E. D.: Servo theory and stuttering. *J. Speech Hearing Dis.*, 25:188-195, 1960.

PENFIELD, W., and ROBERTS, L.: *Speech and Brain Mechanisms*. Princeton, Princeton Univ. Press, 1959.

SHEEHAN, J.: Conflict theory of stuttering. In: *Stuttering: A Symposium*, J. Eisenson, Ed. New York, Harper, 1958.

TOMATIS, A.: *L'oreille et le Language*. Paris, Editions du Seuil, 1963.

TRAVIS, L. E.: The unspeakable feelings of people, with special reference to stuttering. In: *Handbook of Speech Pathology*, L. E. Travis, Ed., New York. Appleton, 1957.

VAN RIPER, C.: *Speech Correction: Principles and Methods*. Englewood Cliffs, Prentice-Hall, 1963.

WEST, R.: An agnostic's speculations about stuttering. In: *Stuttering: A Symposium*, J. Eisenson, Ed. New York, Harper, 1958.

WINGATE, M. E.: Evaluation and stuttering, Part I: Speech characteristics of young children. *J. Speech Hearing Dis.*, 27:106-115, 1962.

APPENDIX

LOGOCYBERNETICS AND BEHAVIOR

THIS APPENDIX will be devoted to making cybernetic speculations about the relationship of oral symbolic behavior to behavior in general. In this regard, Van Riper (1963, Ch. 1) has discussed: (1) speech in thinking, i.e., thinking as a form of inner speech; (2) speech as social control, i.e., speech as a way of controlling the environment and manipulating others; (3) speech as emotional expression, i.e., speech as a way of showing how the speaker feels about himself and others, and (4) speech as self-expression, i.e., speech as a means of self-identification and self-exhibition.

Before entering into the central discussion, which is to associate feedback systems with language and general behavior, a review of selected studies relating to sensory feedback and behavioral mechanisms is in order.

RELATED LITERATURE

Chase *et al.* (1961) investigated differences in individuals in their reactions to delayed auditory feedback as a function of age. Two groups were studied: the age range for one group was four to six years, the age range for the other group was seven to nine years. Under the delayed condition, the older group showed more speech disturbance (rate and syllable prolongation) than did the younger group. The older children were apparently more aware that they were listening to their own voices and more aware of the temporal shift. It was suggested that the greater reaction in the older children might be attributed to their more developed conceptual systems of self and time and their greater awareness of self-produced stimuli (speech), and hence their greater need for unaltered feedback for effective speech monitoring.

The following studies are concerned with the effects of altering the sensory feedback of individuals with behavior disorders.

Goldfarb and Braunstein (1958) reported that schizophrenic children showed less speech disturbance under delayed auditory feedback than did a control group. They revealed that several children in the experimental group identified the delayed voice as belonging to another person. The results suggested a relationship between the effects of delayed feedback and the child's concept of self-identity, and hence it was posited that an advanced development of self-identity and concept function, as might be found in the case of the normal child, would make the child more dependent on unaltered speech feedback for optimal monitoring. The results tend to support the view that schizophrenics as individuals have reduced contact with reality, have less interest in the environment, and have speech which reflects deficiencies in monitoring function.

Different results were found when adult schizophrenics were tested. Sutton, Roehrig and Kramer (1964) reported that the speech of adult schizophrenics is more slowed under the delayed feedback condition than is the speech of normal males, but not more slowed than the speech of normal females. Relative to correct word scores (with reference to misarticulations caused by the experimental condition), the speech of schizophrenics is more affected by delayed feedback than is the speech of normal females, but not more affected than the speech of normal males.

A study which considered the relationships between certain personality variables and reaction to stress in the form of delayed speech feedback was conducted by Spilka (1954). One hundred and fifty college males were studied and it was hypothesized that individuals who showed self-percept stability, paranoid tendencies, and rigidity tendencies would show a greater reaction to the experimental stress condition because of their tendencies to over-react, or to consider external changes important, or to breakdown under stress, than would individuals who showed schizoid tendencies because of their inclination to react more to internal cues. It was found that the most closely related voice variable to such personality functioning was vocal intensity variation.

These studies support the idea that behavior and behavior control are in various ways dependent on sensory feedback mechanisms. The remaining sections of this appendix are concerned with the central purpose of the appendix, namely, a discussion of human behavior and feedback systems.

FEEDBACK SYSTEMS AND NORMAL BEHAVIOR

Automatic control systems have been described in this book as error sensitive, error measuring, self-adjusting, goal-directed systems. The mechanisms that control human behavior may be viewed in a similar fashion, since individuals have the property and potential of being able to adjust their future conduct by virtue of evaluating and of reacting to their past performances. Further, it is believed that the greater portion of human behavior is directed by inner speech activity. That is, individuals direct their overt behavior by telling themselves what to do with covert speech. Finally, adequately functioning behavioral processes may be seen as anti-entropic,* or as processes which generate behavior patterns which decrease confusion and increase order for the individual. Such anti-entropic behavioral feedback systems operate on both intra- and interpersonal levels; descriptions of these two levels follow.

---

* Concept of Gibbs as discussed by Weiner (1954, p. 12).

Intrapersonal. On the intrapersonal level, an individual may prescribe or intend certain ideal behavior, very likely describing it to himself via inner speech, then, by acting he transforms this ideal behavior into actual behavior. Next, he compares his intended behavior, again very likely making the comparison via inner speech, with his actual behavior and makes appropriate behavioral adjustments, when necessary.

When actual and intended behaviors are congruent, and when corrector functions are working efficiently, there should be good personal intracommunication and hence good environmental intercommunication. Following is an example of the operation of this type of intrapersonal behavioral feedback system: Suppose a young man desires to impress a lady friend by exhibiting good manners at a certain social gathering. He may be aware that the young lady is particularly sensitive to good table manners and so he plans to be especially careful in this regard. Before dinner, he may review in his mind, by virtue of inner speech, what ideal eating behavior is and makes plans to act accordingly. During the meal, however, he may become more interested in the good food and less interested about his eating behavior. Suddenly, he reminds himself of his behavioral intentions, evaluates his soup slurping as being less than his intended behavior (negative feedback) and quickly adjusts. Hence, occasionally throughout the dinner, he may inspect his real eating behavior, compare it with the ideal, and continue to make appropriate adjustments for the purpose of moving closer and closer to the ideal behavior; such behavior patterns are anti-entropic or efficient modes since they contribute to an increase in order between himself and his lady friend.

Interpersonal. At least two types of interpersonal behavioral control mechanisms may be recognized. The first type tends to ensure the eliciting by an individual of a certain response from another individual in the environment. The second type involves the awareness by an individual of responses being sought from him by another individual in the environment.

The operation of the first type is observed when an individual seeks a certain response from another individual in the environment, and hence behaves in a certain manner, then evaluates his companion's response, compares the desired response with the actual response and, when necessary, adjusts his behavior in order to bring the desired and actual environmental response into closer approximation. This type of behavioral sensitivity and flexibility is, of course, important to efficient social behavior.

As a specific example of this type of behavioral control, let us return to the young man who is hoping to impress his lady friend. Suppose he has now accompanied his lady friend home and decides to ask man's eternal question to woman; he begins his proposal of marriage and while he continues he very carefully scans her face, posture, and so on, for reactions.

He may have begun with a tough, manly "Hollywood approach" which may run basically like this: Take note of how big and strong and irresistible I am and so let's not waste time, say yes, and let's have done with it. However, he may quickly notice certain negative reactions coming from his lady friend and when he compares her actual response with his hoped for response, he recognizes a substantial error factor and hence decides to quickly adjust his manner of proposal. He now assumes a more loving and gentle attitude and fills the air with sweet romantic phrases. He quickly notes a change in his companion's behavior; she softens and becomes more receptive. Now hoped for and actual responses are in harmony. He finally puts the fateful inquiry to her and, of course, there is an affirmative reply.

The operation of the second type of interpersonal behavioral control involves the awareness by an individual of responses being sought from him by another individual in the environment. In this situation, the individual responds to stimuli generated by a companion, compares his actual response to these stimuli with what he believes is the response being sought by the companion, and makes appropriate behavioral adjustments when necessary, or if he wishes to.

As an illustration of this type of behavioral control, we may once again return to our couple. Once the young lady accepts the proposal, she quickly invites her young swain to inform her father of the good news. Knowing about the father's bias with respect to desired behavior patterns in potential son-in-laws, the young man decides to be forceful and straightforward in his approach. However, upon confrontation with the girl's father, he tenses and becomes anxious and timid. Convinced that the father is seeking a manly type of son-in-law for his daughter and that his present response is not an appropriate one, he firms, makes appropriate behavioral adjustments, and finds himself being congratulated by his future father-in-law.

It should be realized, of course, that in all three examples, the individual might have chosen to behave in an opposite manner if he found his female companion undesirable and wished to disengage himself from her.

In the discussion so far, the reader has recognized the operation of one predominantly internal loop behavioral control mechanism and two forms of predominantly external loop behavioral control mechanisms. When these internal and external loop behavioral control mechanisms are operating efficiently, it is obvious that the individual has a much better chance for more satisfying relationships with society; in other words, his behavior patterns will be anti-entropic or will tend to produce more order in his intrapersonal behavior and hence in his interpersonal behavior. In terms used by de Latil (1957), the described behavioral feedback control mechanisms can be viewed as retroactive systems, that is, part of the effect or behavior feeds back or retroacts upon the cause of the behavior, or the organism, and changes the organism's behavior in certain prescribed ways when it is indicated. The reader should, of course, recognize that the concept of retroactive systems is equal to that of closed loop systems as used in the main body of this book.

FEEDBACK SYSTEMS AND ABNORMAL BEHAVIOR

In contrast, inadequately functioning behavioral processes are entropic, that is, they are processes which generate behavior patterns which increase confusion and decrease order for the individual.

When there is a disturbance in either intrapersonal or interpersonal behavioral feedback processes, there will, of course, be a serious reduction in behavioral efficiency. In feedback terms, the closed loop may be said to have "opened" and hence there is a loss in error-behavior sensitivity and, consequently, in behavioral adjustment processes. With an open loop mechanism, or with the loss or reduction of error-behavior sensitivity and measuring, the young man previously mentioned would not have reacted appropriately to his soup slurping, or to his inappropriate proposal approach to his lady friend, or to his inappropriate image presentation to her father, and, in all cases, he would very likely have suffered negative environmental reactions. Open loop or non-feedback systems have been described by de Latil as interactive systems. Using de Latil's terminology, an interactive system, then, is one where the parts of an organism interact with one another to produce a behavioral effect; however, this effect has no significant effect upon the behavioral mechanisms of the individual. This represents interaction on an intrapersonal level. Interaction on an interpersonal level describes a situation where two individuals interact with one another and where the response of a companion may have no significant effect on the system responsible for the response.

In view of what has been said about efficient and inefficient behavioral patterns and how they may be related to retroactive or interactive behavioral processes, it should be interesting now to discuss possible ways of improving behavioral processes by utilizing concepts generated from feedback theory.

FEEDBACK SYSTEMS AND BEHAVIORAL ADJUSTMENT

It is apparent that in order for an individual to correct certain behavioral deficiencies he should strive to change basically interactive behavioral operations to retroactive operations; that is, it would be important for him to integrate behavioral feedback loops on both the intra- and interpersonal levels. The role of a clinician in this situation would entail the employment of techniques that would help the client to increase his error sensitivity and to improve his error measuring or behavioral comparator functioning and hence his behavioral self-adjustment capacity. Explanations of at least two procedures for strengthening retroactive behavioral operations follow.

Anticipatory Behavioral Feedback. The concept of anticipatory behavioral feedback is related to those servomechanisms which predict the future position of an object, as in the case of a fast moving jet plane, aim the cannon accordingly, and fire the missile at an anticipated location and thereby ensure that target and missile will meet. With respect to behavioral mechanisms, we are referring to the use of synthetic or anticipated experiences as a technique for assisting in closing intrapersonal feedback loops. For example, an individual might be encouraged to imagine a certain scene, such as asking his employer for a raise, to select a certain approach, to consider the characteristics of his employer and, therefore, to imagine the employer's likely response. This type of mental rehearsal might remind the individual that because his employer has certain inclinations, his imagined timid approach would have reduced his chances of receiving the raise. He, therefore, tries another approach which might result in success. Of course, such synthetic experiences do not ensure successful behavior patterns; however, such exercises might very well facilitate the development of increased sensitivity to error behavior.

The reader might respond to the above suggestion by saying that such mental rehearsal is often employed by individuals; however, it is believed that it is not done often enough or in any systematic fashion, nor by all those individuals who might benefit from it. The activity described above represents projected comparing of ideal and actual behaviors and allows for some prior polishing or refining of anticipated behavior.

Informative Behavioral Feedback. Feedback which is generated by actual rather than anticipated behavior is referred to as informative feedback. For example, one step beyond anticipatory feedback is that feedback derived from speaking aloud to an imaginary companion, or that feedback derived from actual rehearsal by the actor, teacher, or speaker. In each of these cases, the individuals may anticipate responses on the basis of their actual performances and make adjustments accordingly. Other activities which contribute to informative behavioral feedback involve techniques which heighten and clarify feedback during actual behavior. At least two ways of doing this will be presented.

Delayed Informative Feedback. In order to provide delayed informative feedback information, an individual may interact with the environment while in the company of a companion who serves as a behavioral shadow or double feedback. That is, after a certain personal interaction has taken place, the companion offers his interpretation of both the subject's behavior and the environmental response. The subject can then compare his version of his intended and actual behaviors and the environmental response with the version of his feedback companion. Similar information can be gained by having motion films or videotape recordings made of certain behaviors such as making a speech, teaching a class, having an argument, and so forth.

Or something a little less elaborate might involve using a body-worn trans-
istorized tape recorder during certain interpersonal relationships such as
having discussions with a spouse, business partners, and so on. These episodes can then be played back and evaluated for behavioral error factors.

Simultaneous Informative Feedback. Accentuating simultaneous informative feedback may be accomplished by performing in front of full length
mirrors or in mirrored rooms for the benefit of increasing visual feedback,
and by speaking while wearing small amplifiers (hearing aid type) for the
benefit of increasing auditory feedback. Such additional informative feedback may eventually contribute to more accurate transformations of desired
into actual performances by sharpening behavioral comparator functions.

In closing, it might be appreciated that, as in the case of speech disorders and speech therapy, the application of the concepts and language of
feedback theory to behavior and its disorders appears interesting and useful.

REFERENCES

CHASE, R. A., SUTTON, S., FIRST, DAPHNE, and ZUBIN, J.: A developmental study
of changes in behavior under delayed auditory feedback. *J. Genet. Psychol.,*
99:101-112, 1961.

DE LATIL, PIERRE: *Thinking by Machine.* Boston, Houghton, 1957.

GOLDFARB, W., and BRAUNSTEIN, P.: Reactions to delayed auditory feedback in
schizophrenic children. In: *Psychopathology of Communication,* P. H. Hoch,
and J. Zubin, Ed., New York, Grune and Stratton, 1958.

SPILKA, B.: Relationships between certain aspects of personality and some vocal
effects of delayed speech feedback. *J. Speech Hearing Dis.,* 19:491-503, 1954.

SUTTON, S., ROEHRIG, W. C., and KRAMER, J.: Delayed auditory feedback of
speech in schizophrenics and normals. Mimeographed report of study supported in part by grants from the National Institute of Neurological Diseases
and Blindness and from the National Institute of Mental Health, 1964.

VAN RIPER, C.: *Speech Correction: Principles and Methods,* 4th Ed. Englewood
Cliffs, Prentice-Hall, 1963.

WIENER, N.: *Cybernetics,* 2nd Ed. New York, Wiley, 1961.

WIENER, N.: *The Human Use of Human Beings,* 2nd Ed. Garden City, Doubleday, 1954.

INDEX

A

Abnormal speech feedbacks
  proprioceptive, 27
  tactile, 27
Actual listener reaction—desired listener reac-
    tion comparison, 19, 41
Actual word product—desired word product
    comparison, 18
After-sensations
  after-hearing, 72, 75
  after-movement, 75
  after-smell, 75
  after-sounds, 72
  after-taste, 75
  after-touch, 75
Alloplastic speech systems, 42
Altered sensory feedback and effects on motor
    behavior
  decreased auditory feedback, 12
  decreased proprioceptive feedback, 12
  decreased tactile feedback, 12
  decreased visual feedback, 12
  delayed auditory feedback, 12
  delayed tactile feedback, 12
  delayed visual feedback, 12
Altered sensory feedback and effects on speech
  accelerated speech feedback, 14
  delayed speech feedback, 14
  synchronous speech feedback, 13-14
Anatomical schema of the speech system, 23
Aphasia, 47
  feedback disturbances, 59
  therapy techniques, 59-60
    body language support, 60
    external loop feedback, 60
    off-setting latency period lags, 60
    internal loop feedback, 60
Arnold, G. E., 63
Articulatory system, 71
  homeostasis, 80
Atkinson, C. J., 14
Audio-phonology, 64
Audioregulation
  in voice therapy, 65-70

additional phonocybernetic therapy tech-
    niques, 69-70
  alteration of voice feedback, 69-70
  imagery voice feedback, 69
  unilateral voice feedback, 69
correct-voice seeking and approximating,
    69
error-voice sensitivity and error voice
    measuring, 67
  comparing error-voice and correct voice
    patterns, 68-69
  establishing the correct voice pattern,
    68
  locating a more efficient voice pattern,
    67-68
re-establishment of appropriate tonal-
    symbol, figure-ground relationship,
    69
reverse tonal-symbol, figure-ground rela-
    tionship, 65-67
of phonation, 63-64
of speech product, 41
Audioverbal loop developmental sequence,
    37-41, 51, 65
Audiovocal loop developmental sequence, 34-
    37, 41, 50, 51, 65, 68, 73
Auditory background, 66
Auditory discrimination, 37, 38
Auditory error signal, 31
Auditory feedback, 13, 14, 39, 64
Auditory figure, 66
Auditory localizing, 35, 71
Auditory masking, 13
Auditory orienting, 71, 73
Auditory searching, 35, 71
Auditory staring, 35, 71
Auditory systems, 64
Autism theory of language development, 41,
    43, 52
Automatic control systems, 5
  closed-loop control, 6, 7, 17, 28
  open-loop control, 6
  psychomotor mechanisms, 9-10
  psychosocial mechanisms, 10-12
Autoplastic speech systems, 42

B

Behavior
feedback systems and abnormal behavior, 103
feedback systems and behavioral adjustment, 103-105
anticipatory behavioral feedback, 104
informative behavioral feedback, 104-105
delayed informative feedback, 104-105
simultaneous informative feedback, 105
feedback systems and normal behavior, 100-103
interpersonal, 101-103
intrapersonal, 101
Berry, Mildred F., 34, 73
Black, J. W., 13, 14, 63
Bloodstein, O., 86, 94
Body English, 55
organized, 55, 60
unorganized, 55
Brain, R., 91
Brain-injured child, 47
minimal, 48
Braunstein, P., 99
Brodnitz, F. S., 63
Brown, G. S., 6

C

Campbell, D. P., 6
Carrier tone, 65
Cerebellum, 26, 27
Chase, R. A., 12, 99
Cherry, C., 95
Closed-loop systems, 6, 7, 17, 28, 76
CNS impairment and language symptoms, 47-48, 50
audition, 47-48
word meanings, 48
words and word arrangement, 48
Concept formation, 48
Conceptual units, 40
Conceptualizing process, 24, 25, 40
Copeland, R. H., 61
Corrector device, 8
speech corrector, 30
Cortico-thalamic unit for speech
Broca's area, 26
supplementary motor area, 26
temporoparietal area, 26
Cybernetics, 5, 10, 64
Cybernetic analogue of the speech system, 22, 77

D

Damping
definition of, 31

overdamped speech system, 31
underdamped speech system, 31, 32, 96
Davis, D. M., 85
de Latil, P., 102
Development of audioverbal loops, 38
Development of audiovocal loops, 36
Developmental dysphasia, 47, 48
Dolch, J. P., 14
Dominant ear, 64, 92
Draegart, G. L., 13, 63

E

Echolalia, 37, 39, 74
Effector unit, 25, 27
generator, 25, 27
modulator, 25, 27
motor, 25, 27
Egocentric language, 39
Eisenson, J., 34, 73
Entropy
anti-entropic therapy techniques, 59-60
oral linguistic entropy, 59
Error-free speech content, 28
Error-free speech product, 28, 77
Error-measuring, 6, 24, 77
Error-sensitive, 6, 8
Error signals, 7, 17, 31
auditory error signal, 31
fluency error signal, 91, 94
therapeutic error signal, 76, 77
zero error signals, 30, 94
Error-sound correction, 77
Error-sound production, 31, 76
Error-sound short circuiting, 80

F

Fairbanks, G., 14, 21, 26, 76
Feedback interpretation of Mowrer's autism theory of speech development, 43
Fulton, J. F., 7

G

Goldfarb, W., 99
Guttmann, N., 14

H

Hagberg, B., 48
Hanley, C. W., 14
Hanley, T. D., 13, 63
Heard word-patterns, 38, 39, 47, 50, 51, 52, 53, 54, 55
Hearing
enriched, 69, 70
Hutton, C., 95

I

Imagery feedback
  mind's articulators, 94
  mind's ear, 55, 69
  mind's eye, 55
  mind's fingers, 55
  imagery looping, 56
  mind's mouth, 55
  mind's nose, 55
Imagination exercise, 11
Information storage
  integrator unit, 24, 25
Ingram, T. T. S., 47, 48
Integrator unit, 23-25
  information storage component, 24, 26, 32
  phase 1 integrator, 24, 26
  phase 2 integrator, 24, 26
  speech content comparator, 25
  speech content corrector, 25
Irwin, J. W., 63, 65, 71, 73, 76, 78
Irwin, O. C., 71

J

Jargon, 38
Johnson, W., 87, 93

K

Kephart, N. C., 12, 34, 40, 48
Kinesthetic monitoring channel, 31
Kirk, S. A., 56
Klein, D., 14
Kramer, J., 100

L

Lalling, 37
Latency period, 51
Latif, I., 55
Lee, B. S., 14
Lehtinen, Laura E., 47, 48
Lewis, R. S., 47, 48
Listener, 44
Luchsinger, R., 63

Mc

McCarthy, J., J., 56
McCroskey, R., 14
McCurry, W. H., 71

M

Maltz, M., 10, 11
Maraist, Jean Ann, 95
Meader, C. L., 20
Mecham, M. J., 34
Metraux, Ruth W., 84
Mowrer, O. H., 41, 42, 50, 52

Muyskens, J. H., 20
Myklebust, H. R., 34
Mysak, E. D., 21, 34, 56, 63, 76, 77, 89, 93

N

Negative feedback, 32
Neologisms, 48

O

Open audioverbal loops, 50
Open audiovocal loops, 49
Open-loop systems, 6
Oral communication, 5
Oral language development
  prepropositional stage, 34-37, 41
    closed internal audiovocal loop, 36-37
    closed internal and external audiovocal
      loops, 37
    open audiovocal loop, 34-35
    closing, internal audiovocal loop, 35-36
  propositional stage, 38-41
    closed, internal audioverbal loop, 39-40
    closed, internal and external audioverbal
      loops, 40-41
    closing, internal audioverbal loop, 38-39
Oral language disturbances in childhood, 49-
  52
  open, internal and external audioverbal
    loops, 50-52
    open, external feedforward and feedback
      audioverbal loops, 52
    open, internal audioverbal loops, 51-52
    open, percept pattern-spoken word pat-
      tern loop, and open, heard word
      pattern-spoken word pattern loops,
      51
    percept pattern-heard word pattern loop,
      50-51
    reciprocal relationship between percept
      pattern and heard-word pattern loop,
      51
  open, internal and external audiovocal loops,
    49-50
Oral language therapy procedures, 52-58
  additional logocybernetic techniques, 57-59
    alloplastic and autoplastic speech charac-
      teristics, 58-59
    double, multiple speech feedback, 58
    regenerative speech feedback, 58
  closing external audioverbal loops, 56-57
    auditory closure activities, 56
    auditory memory span, analysis, and syn-
      thesis, 57
    buildup and breakdown, 57
    definitions, antonyms, and synonyms, 56-
      57

dialogue improvisation, 57
look-do-speak, 57
loop latency period, 57
redundancy and restructuring, 57
verbal assists, 57
verbal associations, 57
closing internal audioverbal loops, 53-56
heard word-patterns, 54-55
loop-closing techniques, 55-56
imagery feedback techniques, 55-56
intraverbalizing activities, 56
percept patterns, 53-54
spoken word-patterns, 55
closing, pleasure sensation-word production
loop, 52-53
Orthophonemic process, 76, 77

P

Penfield, W., 24, 26, 91
Percept formation, 38, 39, 48, 50, 51, 54, 55
Percept pattern, 50, 51, 52, 53
work, 54
Perceptual-conceptual development, 40, 50
Perceptual dysfunctioning, 50, 54
auditory, 51
visual, 50
Perceptual-linguistic development, 38, 51
disturbed, 48
internal loop, 39
Perceptualizing process, 24, 25
development, 40
difficulties, 48
Peters, R. W., 14
Physiological homeostasis, 7
blood pressure regulation, 8
brain rhythms, 9
hormonal balance, 8
respiratory regulation, 8
thermal equilibrium, 7-8
water balance, 8-9
Piaget, J., 39
Positive feedback, 42
Predictor potential for speech, 26
Principle of the unity of the multiple-loop
speech system, 20-21
nonelementalism, 21
relativity, 20
self-reflexiveness, 21
unitary structure, 21
Proprioceptive feedback, 37

R

Rapoport, A., 9
Receptor unit, 21-23
Reflexive vocalization, 35
Respiratory-phonatory-articulatory complex, 26

Ringel, R. L., 14
Roberts, L., 24, 26, 91
Roehrig, W. C., 100
Ruch, T. C., 26

S

Scanning, 9, 65
definition of, 32
interpersonal, 78
intrapersonal, 78
Self-hearing, 35
Self-image psychology, 10, 11
Self-talking, 66
Sensor unit
sensor 1, 27
sensor 2, 27
sensor 3, 27
sensor 4, 27
Servomechanisms, 5 (see also cybernetics, and
automatic control systems) 6, 7, 8, 9,
12
Shearer, W. M., 65
Sheehan, J., 91
Sheridan, Mary D., 34
Smith, K. U., 12
Speaker
lead, 58, 97
slave, 58
Speaking
echo, 94
mirror, 94
slave, 94
Speech
echo, 58
slave, 58
tracker, 97
Speech automaticity, 30, 87, 95
Speech behavior
full cycle of, 34
Speech content, 25, 30, 31
comparator, 25
corrector, 25, 31
monitoring, 31, 41
Speech content corrector, 25, 30
Speech control, 13, 14
Speech development (see oral language development)
facilitation of
alloplastic and autoplastic speech systems,
42-44
regenerative speech feedback techniques,
42
Speech disorders
comprehension, 47
formation, 47
transmission, 47

Speech error infusion, 31
Speech events, 27
Speech feedback, 21
    internal, audioverbal feedback loop, 39, 40, 41
    internal, audiovocal feedback loop, 35, 36, 37
Speech feedback terminology, 28-32
    alloplastic and autoplastic speech systems, 32
    anticipatory speech feedback, 29
    attenuated and amplified speech feedback, 28-29
    double, multiple speech feedback, 29
    infused speech error, 31
    internal and external loop scanning, 32
    positive and negative speech feedback, 28
    regenerative and degenerative speech feedback, 28, 52
    reverse speech feedback, 29-30
    shunted speech feedback, 30
    speech system overdamping and underdamping, 31-32
    steady state and transient speech error, 30-31
    synthetic speech feedback, 29
    zero speech error, 30
Speech feedforward, 21
    environmental, audioverbal feedforward loop, 39, 40
    environmental, audiovocal feedforward loop, 35, 36, 37
    external, audioverbal feedforward loop, 39, 40, 41
    external, audiovocal feedforward loop, 35, 36, 37
Speech fluency, 84
    basal fluency level, 87
Speech formation, 17
Speech model, 36, 37
Speech output, 13
    actual, 30
    corrections of, 30, 31
    desired, 30
Speech pathology, 47
Speech pathology and audiology, field of, 5
Speech product, 13, 30
    disturbances of, 15
    feedback, 30
Speech corrector device, 25, 28
    corrective recycling, 20
    speech product, 29, 30, 80, 82
Speech recycling, 18, 19
Speech scanning, 32

external loop, 32
internal loop, 32
Speech sounds, 47
    acquisition of, 71-73
      auditory approximating, 72
      auditory comparing, 72
      auditory orienting, 71
      auditory scanning, 71-72
      auditory tracking, 72
      speech sound, zero error, 72-73
    irregular acquisition of, 73-76
      irregular approximating, 75
      irregular comparing, 74-75
      irregular orienting and looping, 73
      irregular scanning, 73-74
      irregular, speech-sound zero error, 75-76
      irregular tracking, 74
    therapy for, 76-82
      correct-sound automaticity, 82
      correct-sound seeking and approximating, 80-81
      correct-sound tracking, 81-82
      error-sound measuring, 77-80
        auditory dimension, 78
        tactile-proprioceptive dimension, 79-80
        visual dimension, 78
      error-sound sensitivity, 76-77
      error-sound short circuiting, 80
Speech sound control
    audioregulatory mechanisms, 71, 73
    tactile-proprioceptive mechanisms, 73, 79
Speech sound dimensions
    auditory dimension, 27
    proprioceptive dimension, 27
    tactile dimension, 27
    visual dimension, 27
Speech sound perception, 71, 75
Speech sound production, 71
    standard sound production, 73, 78
Speech sound reception, 13, 71
Speech sound tracking
    auditory tracking, 72
    corrective, 75, 81
    echo tracking, 74
    imagery tracking, 74
    irregular tracking, 74
    slave tracking, 74
Speech system as a closed, multiple-loop system, 17, 30, 32, 34
    anatomical schema of, 23
    cybernetic analogue of, 22, 23, 24
    external loop, 18-19
    ideal system, 32, 58
    internal loop, 17-18, 21-28
Speech system fixation, 32

Speech system oscillation, 32
Speech zero error
  irregular, speech sound zero error, 75
  speech sound zero error, 72
Spilka, B., 100
Spoken word-patterns, 38, 39, 40, 41, 47, 50,
    51, 52, 53, 54, 55
Steer, M. D., 14
Strauss, A. A., 12, 34, 40, 47, 48
Stromsta, C., 63, 64, 92
Stuttering
  developmental, 84, 85
  phases of, 86
Sutton, S., 100
Synthetic experience, 11
Synesthetic stimulation, 54

T

Tactile feedback, 14, 37
Tactile-kinesthetic feedback, 14
Tactile monitoring channel, 31
Tactile-proprioceptive feedback, 29
Tactile-proprioceptive regulation
  speech product, 41
Tactuo-olfactory channels, 54
Teachers College Speech and Hearing Center,
    68
Thought neuronal-pattern, 26
Thought pattern-word pattern comparison, 18,
    41
Thought propagation, 17
Tiffany, W. R., 14
Tomatis, A., 64, 69, 92
Tonal flow
  abnormal, 84
  developmental sequence of, 84-86, 93
  forms of irregular tonal flow, 89-93
    word formation-word production, 91
    word production-anticipation of fluency
      of word production, 91
    word production-listener reaction com-
      parison, 92
    word production-thought pattern com-
      parison, 91-92
    thought pattern-word formation, 90-91
  symptoms of irregular tonal flow, 86-89
    irregular motor reaction, 87-88
      articulatory movements and feedback,
        87-88
      circuit-breaking motor activities and
        feedback, 88
    irregular perceptual-conceptual reactions,
      88-89
      circuit-breaking conceptual activities
        and feedback, 89

misperceptions about intrinsic speech-
    sound difficulty and feedback, 88
therapy procedures for irregular tonal
    flow, 93-97
  diagnosis of type of deautomaticity,
    93-94
  developmental fluency feedback, 95
  re-establish a fluency, zero error signal,
    94-95
    attenuated speech feedback, 95
    solo speech feedback, 94-95
    speaking conditions, 94
    speech imagery feedback, 94
    steady state fluency error signal, 95
  shunted speech feedback, 95-97
    amplified speech feedback, 97
    attenuated speech feedback, 96
    double speech feedback, 97
Tonal generation, 63
Transient speech error, 30
  correction of, 30
Transmitter unit, 25-27
  phase 1 transmitter, 25, 77
  phase 2 transmitter, 25, 77
  speech product comparator, 25
  speech product corrector, 25
  transmission storage, 26
Travis, L. E., 90

V

Van Riper, C., 56, 63, 65, 71, 73, 76, 78, 93, 99
Verbalizing
  automaticity of, 90, 92
  disturbances in automaticity of, 90-93
  processes, 90
Vocalization
  organized, 55, 65, 66
  unorganized, 55, 65
Voice
  control, 63, 64
  disorders, 63
  homeostasis, 69
  leading, 67
  model tone, 65, 66, 69
  pattern, 67-68
    durational dimension, 67
    intensity dimension, 67
    pitch dimension, 67
    quality dimension, 67
  rehabilitation, 63, 64, 65-70

W

Walter, W. G., 9
West, R., 73, 91
Wiener, N., 5, 9

Wingate, M. E., 85
Word approximation, 42
Word-finding difficulty, 48
Word formation, 18
Word neuronal-pattern, 25, 26

Word production, 18
Word product-listener reaction comparison, 19, 41
Word product-thought pattern comparison, 18, 41